To my dearest maybe girl you know how I'm coming for you. The friend that never Judges and always pushes me

Do

The Cancer Slayer
Domenique Mundey

This is a work of nonfiction. However, the author has changed some names, professions, locations, or characteristics of certain people to protect the privacy of those people, as well as the privacy of the author.

Edited by: Jerre Jakee (jerrewrites@yahoo.com) | IG: @jerrewrites | www.authorjjakee.com
Simóne J Banks | IG @ifyoustayedover

Printed in the United States of America
ISBN 978-0-578-81347-9

DEDICATED TO my grandmother Lenora Mundey.

he was born on October 22, 1937 and passed away on September 11, 2002—exactly one year later at 10am when the Twin Towers were attacked—due to ovarian cancer.

She was one of the strongest women I've ever known.

I miss you and I'll love you always.

Love your granddaughter,
Domenique

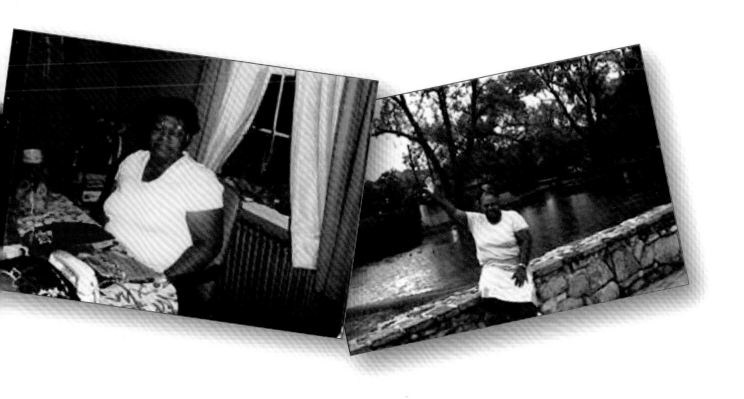

THANK YOU to all of my friends and family who supported, pushed, and held my hand through this entire ordeal. I love you all. Special thanks to all the strangers who reached out and kept me in prayer as well. Also, a special thanks to the following:

Campus Copy Center
3907 Walnut St.
Philadelphia, Pa 19104

Cancer Who Center
3400 Richmond St.
Philadelphia, Pa 19134

Abington Fertility Clinic
1245 Highland Ave. #404
Abington, Pa 19001

HairTrance Hair Boutique
2228 N. Broad St.
Philadelphia Pa 19132

Hair by King
4614 Lancaster Ave.
Philadelphia Pa 19131

The Cancer Slayer

After reading the first few pages of Dom's book I was overwhelmed with emotions!!! Dom baby, you did an excellent job with providing a visual for your readers. Thank you for being so transparent and personable! Thank you for letting us into your life during this traumatic time for you. I feel inspired by your story and I can't wait to read about your transformation in part two.

Love, Shunni

I met Dom just prior to her being diagnosed with cancer and never realized until after reading the draft of her book how much she went through. She is one of the bravest people I have ever met and the most special thing about her is that even when she was going through her lowest time, she was ALWAYS there for me in every way. There is so much more I could say about her, but that being said, she has been an amazing part of my life and I am so happy that she overcame cancer.
I look forward to her friendship for many, many more years to come. I love you Dom and couldn't imagine my life without you in it.

Love, Ron

Table of Contents

Foreword
from David E. Poindexter

From the first time I met this daring and outgoing young lady, Domenique Mundey, I knew that she was about serious business and had a love for family, was compassionate, and more than anything, was one who had a heart to help others. I knew that I was meeting a young lady who was in a league of her own and was charted for greatness and success. Every time thereafter, I would see more and more of how much she cared for people and would put her heart and soul into their lives and apply whatever powers she had to help change the world.

Throughout the years, Domenique has spent her time not only dealing with her own struggles and setbacks but was continually trying to uplift others who were going through the same concerns. She has worked hard to not only give back to others who have dealt with this debilitating disease known as "Cancer", but has worked to raise monies to encourage others to fight the battle, as well as create programs that will raise funds. It's not just that she has gone through this battle sometimes feeling alone, but Domenique has managed to use her faith and talents to "give back".

Domenique's memoir *The Cancer Slayer* totally blew me away because she never showed one ounce of hurt, pain, giving up on life, loneliness, or giving up on her faith to others, including her family. Whenever you would see Domenique in person, you just thought that she was managing and would be alright. From reading this memoir, you will find the struggle and pain that she has gone through daily, as well as long term, and how she battled this disease and kept proving that she would beat this.

There is power and strength in Domenique Mundey's voice; and by this I don't mean loud. Her tone is smooth. It's easy to listen to during her struggles and hardships. All in all, she has found solace in the fact that there is a future that she worked hard to achieve and she plans to fight battles and set goals to move on with her life. Despite the ups and downs, I've seen her at her lowest but she kept on showing this power in her voice by saying that she's going to make it and that "everything is going to be alright". She knew just how to handle her situation, how to describe her pain and the ups and downs that she experienced while dealing with life, her family, and personal relationships, while learning about this disease.

There is power in her message and memoir of her life. The essence of her story is based on her personal life experiences, which are shared in such an intimate fashion that makes you ask questions of how did you make it, why didn't we know, and moreover what does your future look like? As you read, you will picture yourself going along this journey of life's expectancies. While asking yourself how to handle your own hurts and pain, but moreover, how do I move forward and make others believe in themselves, just as Domenique Mundey has done.

May this memoir give you the **"power of hope and encouragement."**

David Poindexter is a retired teacher from the Philadelphia and Cheltenham School Districts. Additionally, Mr. Poindexter taught as a Professor at Community College and Bob Randall Associates (Gratz College). To give back, Mr. Poindexter finds time to manage and promote public speakers throughout the United States, serves on the Board of Global Leadership Academy Charter School, Southeastern Chapter of the Red Cross, Black Male Development Symposium, and Frontiers International. He has also been the recipient of numerous education, civic, and social awards throughout the years. Moreover, he still finds time to mentor those who need a fatherly figure to be a part of their lives and will never stop "giving back". He has a Bachelors Degree in Elementary Education and Masters in Special Education from Antioch University.

Preface

Have you ever had an out-of-body experience? Have you ever had to legitimately fight for your life over something so surreal and so traumatic, that it stays with you years after? Have you ever looked death in its eyes?

Some of us can say that we have because we were in the wrong place at the wrong time or in other cases, right where we needed to be. I have always lived by the quote, "everything happens for a reason". For me, thinking that way played a significant part whenever I consider why and what I had to go through. I think that's why I was able to handle my situation as gracefully as I did.

Before learning I had cancer, I didn't have any of the apparent symptoms; I wasn't "sick" and I didn't look "sick". I learned later that fatigue is the primary symptom of breast cancer. I still don't know if having breast cancer was the reason, or if I was tired and just over-worked. Unfortunately, they don't have an app for that!

I contemplated writing this so I would have the opportunity for my narrative to reach people further than social media. During my journey, I amplified a more extensive audience by way of social media. I'm calling my story *The Cancer Slayer* because of how I approached my situation. I decided to share my story with the hope to bring awareness to society by demonstrating and clarifying what I did to help myself.

With the material I provide, I hope to show everyone how to fight cancer as stress-free and confident as possible. Hopefully, after reading my book, you can help someone or use the information for yourself. So many folks expressed how much I inspired them with my story. I only want to inspire and do so long after my fight is over.

I never thought I would be able to write a book. I never thought I could be an author. Things seem so out of reach. So unachievable in this world. People like me aren't authors. But, then again, I thought people like me don't get cancer either.

WHO

AM

I?

My name is Domenique. I am an adventurous, social butterfly and I love meeting new people and exploring new places. Especially here in my hometown of Philadelphia, PA or sometimes even out of town. For the most part I'm optimistic, but I have my moments just like everyone else. At the time I was diagnosed, I was a healthy 30-year-old. I didn't do any recreational drugs or engage in any risky behaviors.

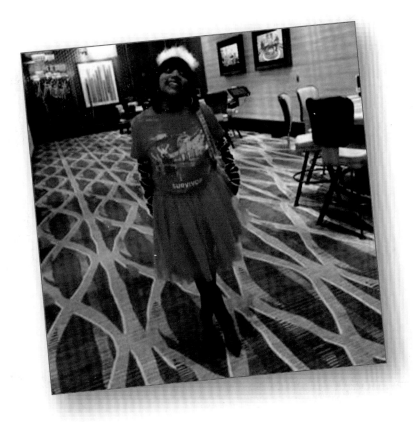

I smoked hookah and drank alcohol socially. I was at the very end of a long-term relationship

I didn't do recreational drugs or engage in any risky behaviors.

with a man whom I thought I was going to marry. After accepting that we were probably not going to reconcile, I started focusing on my future. I started taking prerequisite classes for nursing; took a short break to obtain a CNA certification expecting to be enrolled back in classes the upcoming semester. All of that was happening at the same time I hired a realtor to help me commence the house-hunting process. Little did I know that my world, and everything I knew and was working on, was about to come to a halt in just a matter of a few weeks.

THE
BEGINNING

It was November, a few weeks before my 30th birthday, and I was planning a big party for my friends and family. I was finalizing the last little details and was with my friend, Marcus, as I usually was on most Sundays. Either he was at my house or me at his, watching our show *The Walking Dead*. After our show ended, we had our own little session of "The Talking Dead". We said our goodbyes and set our date for the following week—same time, same place.

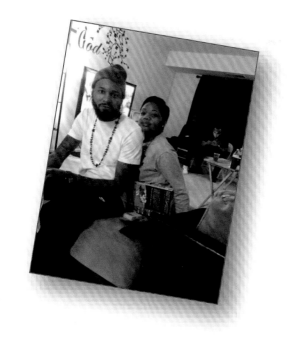

I met Marcus at TGIFriday's many years ago with an old friend. I remember thinking, "Wow, he's handsome." I had never really been into light-skin men. So, I just cracked jokes about him being light-skin and played out. We laughed the entire time. I don't recall exactly what I was saying because I was drinking, but I'm sure it was some wild stuff. I can only imagine how he perceived me back then. We sat there for some time joking and laughing. He thought I was dope, so we exchanged numbers and kept in touch.

Anyway, that Sunday, I don't know why, but he gave me a bearhug and lifted me from the floor while doing so. I felt some pressure on the right side of my chest in the breast area. There was no pain, just a little pressure and a significant sized lump. I had him feel it as well.

He snatched his hand back swiftly and said, "Yo! You should get that checked out dog." I had very little concern considering I had never been sick or hospitalized. In any case, I still scheduled an appointment to see my primary doctor the week before my party. I continued with preparing for my birthday party and doing my routine.

I was running behind schedule! However, when I arrived at my doctor's office, to my surprise, she wasn't there. It slipped my mind that she relocated. Consequently, I missed my appointment and would have to reschedule. The next date wouldn't be until the week following my party. Due to my health concerns and her better judgment, she squeezed me in.

Years prior to this appointment, I had a thin, milky discharge from my breast when they were stimulated. The doctor prescribed me vitamin D to take once a week for this. Taking the vitamin D resolved my issue; and I learned that I was vitamin D deficient.

During my exam, she did the routine tasks: blood pressure, temperature, etc. Then she did a breast exam. After feeling the two lumps I thought were one, she grew more interested in the masses in question. When I left my appointment, I had a prescription for a Bilateral Mammogram and Breast Ultrasound even though I was younger than the standard age to require them.

When I attempted to schedule my exams at Einstein Hospital, there were no appointments for about a month and a half out. I accepted the date but was unsatisfied with the lack of urgency the hospital had for my health. There was a cap on my insurance, which meant that any doctor I saw had to be within the network of my primary doctor. That said, I either went to Einstein, or I would have been financially liable for my visits 100%.

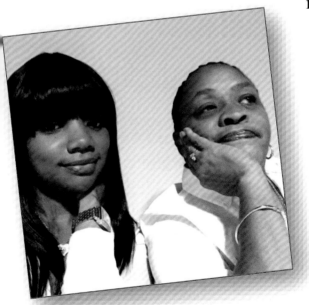

I told my mother, Kimberly, how far out my upcoming appointment was and she was appalled. She called them and told them that it was unacceptable and threatened to call the local news stations. That is my mother's "go-to threat" when dealing with businesses. When I talked to my mom again, my appointment was the following week, a few days before my birthday.

My mom is just a bit taller than me but acts as tall as Shaq. She's outspoken and has a great sense of humor. However, she doesn't play much when it comes to her kids. She got hurt on her job many years ago and needed limited to extensive assistance with many things around the house. In the beginning, it was hard for her. But, currently, she accepts that her children must help her as she did for us when we were younger.

After all my mom did for my appointment to be scheduled sooner, would you believe I confused it with my dentist appointment? Luckily, my mother left a lasting impression on them; my next date was just two days after my birthday.

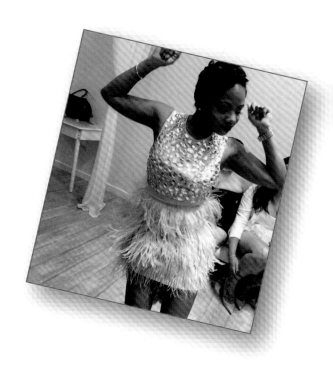

The day of my party was here. My mother and I prepared all the food. We had potato salad, string beans, meatballs, chicken wings, etc. and I had a dessert table catered. I didn't have anything that I didn't enjoy. I found myself stealing the cupcake pops my guests had put down with thoughts of enjoying them later. Nearly everyone I invited was in attendance. It was a night to remember; nothing short of amazing.

India, a friend of mine whose mother had recently passed away surprised me and stopped by. I hadn't expected her to come, but she managed to pull herself together so she could attend. I had never lost a parent, so I didn't know how India felt or what to say. I just tried to be there the best I knew how. Due to my new health concerns, I couldn't bring myself to attend her mother's funeral. I was questioning my own fate and felt too afraid to see a corpse. I do believe she felt someway about my decision not to show up. But we don't speak about it. It's never been an easy topic to talk about, but I believe she forgives me.

Two days later, I arrived on time for my appointment and was feeling optimistic. I heard my name called, and I went back into another room where other women were already in their gowns and waiting to have their mammograms.

My name was eventually called again, and I went into the examination room. The machine looked a bit different than an ordinary x-ray machine or how I imagined them to look. It was tall and my body didn't go inside. I stood very close in front of the x-ray machine. I placed my right breast in between the two plates of the device, with my arm on the side. The plates firmly pressed against my right breast until it was as flat as possible. There was a considerable amount of pressure and discomfort but no pain. I had images taken from a few different angles, which lasted about 10-15 minutes.

A few moments later, the ultrasound technician came and escorted me back to my room for my next exam. As talkative as I am, I had a million questions:

"How will you know if it's cancer? What will it look like?"

The tech seemed focused, as her responses were short. So, I figured I should be quiet and let her finish her job. When she was complete, she excused herself.

I couldn't believe my ears. I was sick.

She returned with a doctor, and they both concentrated hard while reviewing the images. I began to get a bit nervous but remained quiet. They discussed what they were looking at amongst themselves. I tried to ear hustle but couldn't hear well enough.

Then, they both turned around simultaneously and asked, "Ms. Mundey, are you here alone?" At that moment, seeing the concern in their faces, I felt my heart in the pit of my stomach.

"Yes, yes, I'm alone," I said, eager to learn what they had to say.
"Ms. Mundey, I'm sorry, but I suspect this to be cancer."

I couldn't believe my ears. I was sick. I couldn't believe I had taken the situation so lightly that now I was in the hospital, crying my eyes out with two strangers.

It was a long walk back to the dressing room. My mind was racing, and I was shaking as if I had Parkinson's disease. I was lost in a daze. I hadn't known what "lost in a daze" felt like until that day. I was walking, but I didn't see myself moving away or closer to my destination. My ears were clear, but I couldn't hear the people chattering in the waiting room. The technician talked to me the whole way to the dressing room, but I hadn't heard one word, she said.

While waiting for my car at the valet, I felt dirty; like everyone knew I had cancer and was judging me. It was a similar feeling to when I contracted a sexually transmitted disease for the first time. I felt disgusting. Looking back now, I know how much different this was. That was something I couldn't avoid. Learning I had cancer had nothing to do with who I dated.

I felt my tears drying swiftly as the cold winter air hit my face. I called and delivered the news to my mom, and she went off. She said the doctors couldn't give me an "almost diagnosis", and they still had to do other tests to confirm that it was, in fact, cancer. She insisted that I relax until I had further testing done. I can't lie; her words made me feel a little better. I can't say that I felt great, but I would be able to sleep that night.

When I got home, my mom was pacing the floor, still furious about the way the doctor delivered the information. I'm sure part of that was her fear of the worst. She tried to reassure me that the news wasn't definite. She also advised me to keep busy and continue to work on the things I was working on to keep my mind occupied.

I had never been a very spiritual person, but that night I prayed really, really hard. I thought to myself, "I'm a nice person. I don't do things with malice, this type of stuff should be happening to the people who are malicious or just evil in general like killers, rapists, etc. They needed to be punished and taught a lesson. Not me. I'm very humble, so I know for sure I don't deserve this. I'll be fine."

The next day, I didn't have to call anyone if I knew my mom. News spread like wildfire and everyone found out. Before I knew it, my phone was ringing back to back. Instead of answering it, I let it go to voicemail. What my mom said continuously replayed in my head, "That was so unprofessional! You still have to have other tests done. It has to be a solid confirmation".

I thought to myself, "I've always been healthy." I mean, I smoked hookah, but that couldn't give me breast cancer. Could it? My mind was going a mile a minute. Did I jeopardize my health? Like when I used those soaps, lotions, powders, etc. Even though I saw that commercials that implied that they were cancer causing. The same things that I continued to use/do without any regard or concerns. I never used recreational drugs either. I mean, I experimented with weed (I hated it). But that was it. There were many benefits to ingesting marijuana, even though I don't consider it a harmful recreational drug.

After seeing Dr. Zimmerman, an oncologist at Fox Chase Cancer Center, to discuss my results, I learned that there were four masses in my right breast. Instead of the two. They ranged from 1.2-2.2 cm. He suggested that I get a biopsy guided by ultrasound. A biopsy is when a small needle is used to take a sample of the tissue in question. The sample is sent out to be reviewed and analyzed. This biopsy would confirm if I had cancer or not.

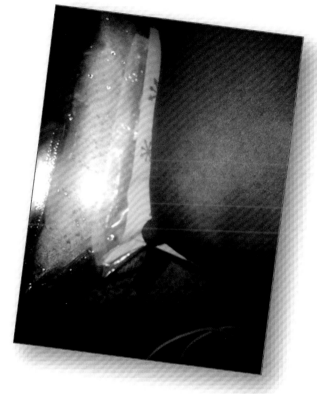

I was still nervous, but confident, for the most part. This time I came prepared. I had the gang with me: my mother, father, brother, and my girlfriend Kee. I went back and hopped onto the examination table.

They used some Lidocaine to numb the area they would be accessing for the samples. They placed each sample in test tubes. Also, metal clips were placed over the masses in case they were cancerous, to be easily removed during surgery. The procedure was simple, and there was no downtime required.

Now, I just had to go home and continue with my life while I waited for my results. It was a Monday, and I had until Thursday.

WHAT'S IT GOING TO BE?

W aiting for my results was like waiting for an AIDS/HIV test after a long summer of being a loose woman. It was a LONG three days. However, Thursday came and went with no call from the doctor. Most of the doctors I've met say, "no news is good news." So, I went out Thursday night, to the neighborhood bar, and drank like a fish with my mom and brother. I had to catch my dad the next day; it was a work night. I celebrated because I knew that they had made a mistake. It wasn't cancer, but something else. Everyone in the bar I knew turned up with me as well. I had a good time. I was able to enjoy myself for the first time in weeks. I wasn't even concerned with what it could be, because if it weren't cancer, anything else was manageable.

The next day I shared the good news on social media and went in for an overtime shift. I was geeked up, knowing that I had done all that worrying for no reason. God was so good. My phone was ringing off the hook again with so many different numbers. Just friends and family were reaching out, congratulating me, and spreading love and warm wishes. After lunch, a (215) 214 number called, and without hesitation, I answered the phone.

Waiting for my results was like waiting for an AIDS/HIV test.

Me: Hello?
Caller: Yes, this is doctor so-and-so. I'm calling from Fox Chase Cancer Center. Can I speak to Ms. Domenique Mundey?

Me: This is she!
Caller: I'm calling to discuss your biopsy results. When do you think you would have time to come in and discuss them?

Me: I'd rather discuss them over the phone. I'm tired of doctor's appointments, and I don't want to come in for something that you can tell me over the phone.

Caller: We usually require our patients to come in to confer about results, but I guess we can talk over the phone this one-time, Ms. Mundey.

She spoke for a few minutes speaking fluent medical jabberwocky. I couldn't comprehend much, but I listened anyway. Then, she said:

Caller: I'm sorry, Ms. Mundcy, but the cells were cancerous.

Me: I'm sorry. What exactly is cancerous? Does that mean they could cause cancer? You don't have to be sorry I'm just grateful we caught it in time.

Caller: No, Ms. Mundey, What I mean is the cells determined that you have breast cancer.

I started to grow angry.

Me: How could everyone there drop the ball? Why didn't anyone call me to tell me yesterday? I was supposed to get a call yesterday! You don't understand how hard I celebrated yesterday, all because you all didn't call me. (Hell, I was still hung over from celebrating the night before). After celebrating not having cancer, you're now calling me telling me that I do have a disease.

Words could never express how I truly felt at that moment. I was more than devastated.

The first thing I thought was, "Omg! Am I going to die?"

The first thing I thought was, "Omg! Am I going to die?" Then, "Is my hair going to fall out?" I couldn't believe that after all the testing and waiting that I was sick in real life. I had cancer. How could I have cancer? I looked and felt fine. It was the hardest pill I ever had to swallow—well, the second hardest pill. The first was Flagyl for bacterial vaginosis.

I called Marcus to tell him what the doctor said. He was deeply saddened. He had been checking on me daily, but I didn't have any solid information until now. Then I called my ex and I told him. He responded telling me he was sad, and heart broken. After that, I called the guy I was dealing with at the time, but he didn't answer. Then, I called my mom. I know that order seemed off but, that's just the way it went. My mom assured me that everything would be ok. I could hear the funk in her voice as she talked to me, "I love you, and you are so strong. You will get through this, I promise," she said. I told her I would call her back. I needed to call my dad.

After I delivered the news, his mind and heart filled with disbelief and heartache. I could tell he was upset. I could hear it in his voice, and he just kept saying, "damn." He must have said it about 13 times. I guess at a time like that, what else could he say? I sent out a text to my friends and family and asked them not to share it with anyone because I didn't want anyone to know, although I had shared my journey on social media up until this point. The truth is, I was embarrassed, and I also didn't want people looking and treating me different.

At first, I called for emergency relief. I wanted to go home! Not too long after, I changed my mind. I figured I'd been working all this time, not even knowing I was sick. So, why leave and miss money to go home, lay down, and be miserable? Of course, my mother wanted me to leave. But **"I'm not a quitter"** quickly became my thought. I chose to live by those words.

About an hour later, my mother and father were at my job with my dog, Toby. I was probably the most excited to see him. You would have to have a dog to understand that kind of love. Toby was a gift from my ex. He wasn't half as attached to him as I was. So, when we separated, I took him. That's my son. We stood outside, and we cried for a little while. That was only my second time seeing my dad cry in my life. The first time was at his mother's funeral years ago. Not too long after, I went back inside to complete my shift.

I didn't want to give my life to cancer. I wanted to live my life while fighting cancer.

That day, I decided that I would continue to work and do anything I wanted to do if I could. But, if I weren't up for it, then I wouldn't. I didn't want to give my life to cancer. I wanted to live my life while fighting cancer. I wanted to continue to push towards my goals and be able to have money to do anything my heart desired, all the while fighting cancer.

A series of scans had to be conducted to determine staging before any treatment could be provided. I also needed to decide where I wanted to receive treatment. First, I had a CT scan of the chest, pelvis, and abdomen. I think back to having to drink a disgusting thick, white contrast called Readi Cat (Barium Sulfate Suspension) to prepare for the scan. Years later and I still gag at the thought of having to drink it.

Upon my arrival I filled out a questionnaire which was protocol to provide some knowledge about my health background. I changed into my gown and went to have my scan completed. The machine was big with a hole in the middle, and a narrow table in front of it. I laid on the table, and then I had an IV put in my arm. After she explained what would happen, she stepped out of the room to begin the test.

The table I was lying on slid into the machine. It made a low buzzing noise while capturing images. The exam was almost complete when the tech came back and injected a special dye in my IV. "Your whole body is going to get warm, but don't panic; it is completely normal." I felt my body warming up quickly, but it wasn't HOT. A few minutes after, I was done and free to go.

Later, the images revealed a questionable lesion on my liver that was thought to be Focal Nodular Hyperplasia or FNH. I needed a further review but, it wasn't that crucial because it didn't reveal any metastasis.

Following that, I had a bilateral breast MRI. I arrived and repeated the steps like all the other exams. After a while, I didn't even need people to tell me what I needed to do because it was repetitive. I had to lie back on a slim table that slid back partially into the machine. I placed my earphones on my ears to listen to music to tune out the loud sound of the engine; it didn't help much, though. This machine was massive, just like the one for the CT scan, but it was loud as it took pictures of the inside of my breast. The procedure lasted about 50 minutes. These images had to be reviewed and analyzed, as well.

I chose to have the My Risk BRCA analysis performed. BRCA is optional, and some insurance companies do not cover this because it is not necessary. It is a blood test that utilizes DNA analysis to see if there are significant mutations in your genes.

I waited two weeks, there were insufficient amounts of data to determine if there was an increased amount of risk for cancer in my cells. The results were inconclusive, which is one of the possibilities. **BUMMER!** However, I would still consider taking preventative measures just in case.

> *However, I would still consider taking preventative measures just in case.*

That same day I had a bone scan. I received an injection of a radioactive substance. Then, I was allowed some time to get something to eat while allowing the element to work its way through my bloodstream. When I returned, I had to lie still on a slim table yet again. However, this machine had two large plates that circled the table around my body. The procedure lasted for about an hour.

After completing all the necessary scans, the mass, including a lymph node under my arm, were positive for cancer. Ultimately, the staging was an aggressive invasive ductal carcinoma and metastatic adenocarcinoma grade 3. My diagnosis was complex because my lymph node was her2 positive; however, my breast was her2 negative. It was also Er positive and Pr variable.

Er and Pr are receptors found in breast cancer. If either of these receptors is present, then they are considered positive, and if they aren't, then, of course, they would be negative. It is possible to have one of each receptor. Although most receptors are negative or positive, it is also possible for a receptor to be variable, which means it is part of both.

LET'S GET READY TO RUMBLE!

Over the next few weeks, I mapped out my plan. I needed to make specific changes to fight my battle as easily and happily as possible. After all, this was no ordinary fight. This fight was not a breakup with my spouse and dealing with my emotions. This was not an argument with my girlfriend. This was legit a fight for my life; losing was not an option.

One decision I made was to cut anything and everything out of my life that caused me stress and pain. Anything that brought me negative vibes had to go. I needed my mind frame to be positive and healthy.

I was still arguing with my ex about our relationship, which was over. We weren't doing much besides accusing each other of messing with other people and denying it to one another. All while we were dealing with other people. That had to end.

I had to accept that I wouldn't be taking classes that upcoming semester. Assuming I wouldn't be able to attend class between doctor appointments, suffering from symptoms, and work. I contacted the realtor and told her why I had to conclude house hunting for a while. Not being able to begin the house-hunting process was hurtful. However, turning down the job at a reputable hospital hurt me the most; so much that I'm just sharing it. I didn't want to talk about it. I had been looking for a new job for quite a while, and now I had one of the most desirable offers on the table and I couldn't take it. Because company policy was that I couldn't apply for intermittent leave until after being on the job for 12 months, and this was my first-time battling cancer, I had no idea what to expect.

I had to cut anything and everything out of my life that was causing me stress.

I chose to put my energy into doing everything that would put me in a better position. I figured I would still do what I could to work towards my goals in other ways. One goal was to continue to improve my credit score. That way, when I was ready to buy a house again, I could get the best rate possible. I did what I could to make myself more comfortable in my mom's house. I took all of my stuff out of boxes and tried to stay ahead with most of my tasks.

When I learned that some insurance plans pay for wigs, I jumped right on it. I got a prescription for a cranial prosthesis from my oncologist. I started to make the appropriate calls. I called my insurance company to see if they honored prescriptions for wigs. I wanted them to pay for the entire unit, but I had to be satisfied with the 50% reimbursement. Hey! It was better than nothing. Next, I checked the prosthetic store in the Fox Chase Cancer Center. I walked past the store so many times but never went inside even though I knew they had wigs there.

I was disgusted with their selection of wigs. To my surprise, none of the wigs seemed to be for African Americans. All the wigs and hairpieces seemed to be for Caucasian and/or Asian women and men. That was very

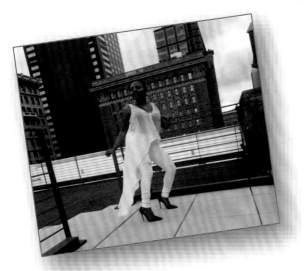

discouraging and disappointing. However, I didn't let that get the best of me. I spoke with someone at the cancer center, and they gave me some names of some other places that had wigs specifically for cancer patients. I received a recommendation for Wig a Doo. That place didn't have anything to accommodate me either. At this point, I was convinced that the same people owned these places. They had no updated wigs. I wasn't trying any more of these places.

Luckily for me, wigs had come a long way since back in the day. For one, wigs were now called units, and they were well liked because of their convenience and versatility. Lace frontals and closures can be customized to match your complexion, so the hair appears to be coming out of your scalp. They were the most realistic units I had ever seen in my life, like the ones Beyoncé wears.

I called my friend Ivory and told her we were going to Baltimore to get some hair. She was always down for a good road trip, anyway. The unit I wanted was about $500 dollars. So, I had to put my hands on it before I purchased it. When we got there, the hair was more than I reckoned it to be. We bought everything we wanted and spent well over $1000 each. Nonetheless, we were happy with our purchases, and it was worth the 2.5-hour ride.

I hit a snag when I called to have my funds reimbursed, though. I found that in fact my insurance company didn't honor prescriptions for units. But after reviewing a recorded call I had with them, they had to show me the money.

After accepting what was reality, I decided I would share my condition with everyone on social media. I don't know what I expected the responses to be, but they were very warm, empathetic, and sympathetic. Many people shared many words of sympathy, encouragement, faith, and prayer. Although I knew my friends and family would support me, I realized that I would receive a greater amount of support from my followers and some complete strangers.

... On social media, everyone becomes a doctor.

One con about sharing on social media is that everyone becomes a doctor. Everyone started recommending a change of diet. The one I heard most was to stop eating red meat. Another was to have an alkaline based diet and eat organic and add sour sop to my diet. I was also told to leave my support system here and go to Honduras to see Dr. Sebi. The list only continued! It got so overwhelming that at times I would deactivate my page. I would have so many personal issues going on and then someone would come and say, *Hey, my mom died from cancer after fighting for so long; keep fighting though.*

I didn't understand how anyone could think that a statement like that would be motivating in any type of way. It never made sense to me. If anything, it was discouraging me more than anything. I would think, "Am I doing this for nothing, if I'm going to die anyway?" But I understand that they were trying to encourage me.

A few people told me to go to a young lady's page named Nadirah. She was a cancer survivor who shared her story. They told me that her page would give me some inspiration and it did. A friend of mine, B, made sure I was in direct contact with her.

After looking through her page, I learned a few things about her. She was a few years older than me and had been in remission a few years at that time. She had lymphoma cancer and a beautiful daughter who looked just like her. Most of all, she won her battle, and she was beautiful. Even after having some of the symptoms I would soon face, she was back to living her life. With that, I said if she could do it so can I. I remember a picture she posted. It stuck with me until this day. She had on a long, green kimono type of cover up. It seemed to be flowing in the wind. Her hair was full and well-manicured. I thought to myself, "I will be myself again after all of this."

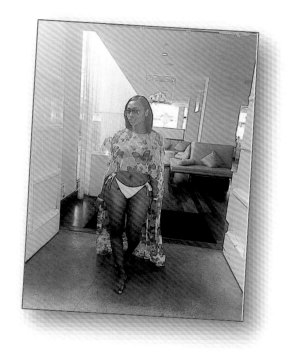

When I talked to her, she was very welcoming. We talked about quite a few things including how her battle went. She also told me I would have my good days and my bad days. She told me that my biggest supporters would most likely be complete strangers. She said that I needed to get rid of the negative energy I had around me for my battle to be successful. Lastly, she told me I would for sure lose some friends, but I would also build some unbreakable bonds. I took in and accepted all that she had told me. She gave me permission to contact her with any questions, or concerns I had. Even if I just wanted to talk and I did. I could never thank B enough for connecting me to Nadirah.

Briefly after sharing with my social media followers, Penelope suggested she make a GoFundMe account for me. Penelope is my childhood girlfriend. I call her "P." She's one of my besties. We have been friends for over 20 years. She always has my back, and she'll check me whenever I'm on some bull crap, quick. But, for the most part, she's always on my side. You only meet friends like her once in a lifetime, twice if you're lucky enough. Lucky for me, I've had her all these years.

Anyway, I was totally against the GoFundMe. I didn't want people to think I was begging. I worked, and I had beautiful things, so I figured no one would want to help me financially, assuming I had it all. I've seen GoFundMe accounts before, and I have even

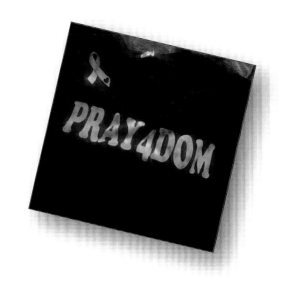

donated to quite a few. I just didn't wish to have one of my own. After all, I didn't think I needed one for myself. How much could the co-pays be?

My co-pays had never been astronomical before, and even though this situation was different, I didn't know if it would be that bad. Little did I know the bills were piling up already, and I hadn't even started treatment yet. I got a few people's opinions, and they all suggested I move forward and set up an account because I may not be able to work like I was used to or at all. So, as a result, I changed my mind and allowed P to set up a GoFundMe for me. Mine was www.helpdombcancerfree.com. It started to raise funds faster than I expected with a goal of $15,000. It gave me great liberation, knowing people wanted to support me. It wasn't the funds that I was happy about; it was knowing people cared enough to try to assist me.

However, after announcing my GoFundMe, I was in the hair salon when I saw someone I knew. We had small talk and then she mentioned that a friend of hers asked her why I didn't just sell some of my material things to raise money. I couldn't believe how insensitive people could be. That's another one of the cons when you share your life on social media.

Soon after, an associate of mine, Keisha got some shirts made and sold them for me. The material and the screening were rich. She purchased crew neck as well as a "v" neck. However, they were more expensive. I needed more of a profit and did some research for other people who did screen-printing. I discovered that DJ GM, a popular DJ here in Philly had a screening company. After going over the numbers, I would be profiting about 70% vs. 40 % per shirt. So, I placed an order for an abundance of shirts, and I was so overwhelmed with t-shirt sales I had a t-shirt drive that upcoming Tuesday.

I requested that everyone who wished to purchase a shirt meet me at The Clubhouse on Broad St. Woah! I was shocked by the support. I had quite a few boxes of shirts; I sold out and had to order more. I gave receipts to the guests who made purchases but had to wait until the next batch was available. B brought his friends, and they bought everything

I had and some. I couldn't have been more appreciative for all the continuous support from my friends, family, and followers.

BET
IT
ALL
ON
YOURSELF

A fter seeing how well the shirts did, my friends proposed that I have a fish fry. I thought about it, and I was still against it. I figured people had bought my shirts and donated to my go-fund-me. I didn't see them coming to a fish fry to spend another $15 dollars. I thought it felt greedy. Besides, whenever I have an event, my anxiety gets the best of me. I'm constantly dreading lousy weather or a complete flop. So, I rarely have them unless they are intimate. After all, I was already more than grateful for the money I had raised thus far. However, my friends managed to convince me again to **bet it all on myself**.

I went for it. My friend SL created my tickets and formatted them to a PDF form. My friend Nor who owned a copy center offered to print my tickets. When I picked them up, they were top of the line, ok! They even had a precut line where they would rip as tickets.

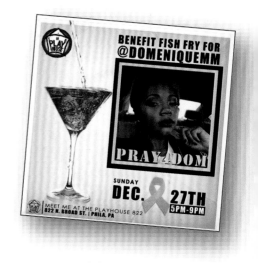

I got straight to business. So many people bought tickets and supported in many different types of ways. There were so many people helping me sell tickets; it was hard to keep track. Things were looking good. The day of my fish fry, I felt like everything that could go wrong did. The forecast said rain, my biggest fear. Secondly, the venue that I was set to have my fish fry at, which was the same place I sold my shirts at, seemed to have all these additional fees mentioned the day of the event and not during the initial conversation. I had to pay for security, and I had to pay for the DJ, etc. All these things would have been fine, but I had never had a fish fry before and felt that mentioning it to me last minute was unprofessional. I thought they were trying to take advantage of me because I was ignorant about how these events worked. That may have not been the case but, that's why it's vital to force contracts. Taking people's words can cause too much confusion because things are unclear. Consequently, at the last minute I decided to change venues.

My first option was the BJ club, which was a couple of doors down from the Clubhouse. I would still have a prime location. Unfortunately, the BJ club didn't operate on Sundays. Sunday was probably his day to relax. I needed a master plan to convince him to open for business. I started utilizing "my connects". I called my girlfriend Kendall first. She worked for Bruce, the owner. So, I figured she would have the best chance of convincing him to open for business. I had a few other people who were current employees, and former employees call as well. I needed them all to back me on this one. At first, he said no, because he liked things to be a certain way. After some more begging, he agreed to open the BJ Club.

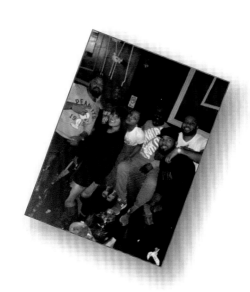

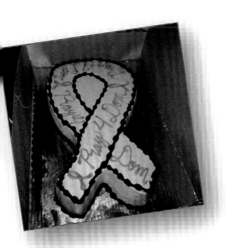

After talking over the numbers and giving him the grand total of tickets sold thus far, I only had to pick up some fish to make sure we had more than enough. I still feared that it would be a dud, but it was in full motion at this point, unless I wanted to spend the next twelve months trying to refund people their money. Thus, no matter the outcome, I just wanted to enjoy myself. I dropped the fish off and went to get myself together for my event.

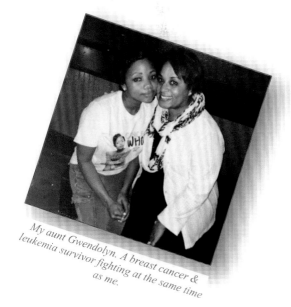

My aunt Gwendolyn. A breast cancer & leukemia survivor fighting at the same time as me.

I was running tardy, as usual. To my surprise, upon my late arrival, many people were already there. P was at the door, taking money and tickets. I also noticed "Pray for Dom" bracelets guests could purchase and breast cancer pins that my girlfriend Liah brought for me to sell. Most of my family is punctual, so they were there already enjoying themselves. Then, it started raining and then it poured. I was so upset. I wanted to cry. I was sure nobody else was coming. However, people continued to flood in. Before I knew it, all three floors were open, and I was having the time of my life.

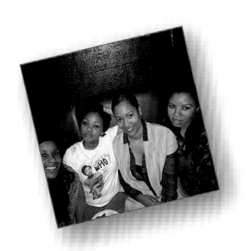

While taking pictures with everyone, I began questioning why they had all come. Were they just there to take pictures in case I died? Were they there just to "do it for the gram?" A lot of people will come around because it's what everyone else is doing, or it's negative (misery loves company). However, it's a different crowd when it's something positive. Have you ever thought about how fast a lousy rumor circulates compared to something positive? It's kind of like that. Or that could have been my mind again since quite a few people told me all the support was "fake love."

The amount of support I had was unforeseen. Having just one bartender wasn't even enough to supply the demand for drinks. Bruce asked around to hire another one. Some people were having too much fun to work; others were unprepared to work. Finally, he was able to find someone to work, and she got to work and earned hundreds in tips that night.

On top of that, my guest had cleaned the kitchen out. Bruce did his best to make sure everyone had something to consume. When the food for the fish fry ran out, he used his food. Some people had shrimp and chicken, and others had chicken tenders and fish along with fries. I couldn't have been more pleased with his customer service and commitments to making sure my guests were satisfied.

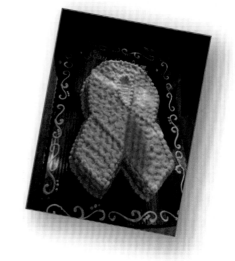

Before I knew it, 9 p.m. presented itself. It was time for everyone to depart, but despite everyone having to work the next day, Bruce allowed the party to continue. At the very end, I had two beautiful breast cancer cakes that my friends K and Liah purchased for me.

My total was over $6,000 dollars. I deposited that into my go-fund-me account. I later regretted that because they take a percentage of each donation, and another portion goes to "WePay" for each check they send out. Nevertheless, the fish fry was a success.

As they say, **"self-doubt is your biggest obstacle."**

As I mentioned before, I was at the end of a long-term relationship. Before my fish fry, I didn't feel like Hass was being as supportive as I expected him to be. I felt like all things considered; he should have at least made me one of his prime concerns on his list of things to do. It was causing me to be distressed. My expectations weren't met, and I was very disappointed. So, I stopped answering his calls and I ignored his texts. I'd rather ignore him, than continue to be let down. I guess he got the hint because, at my t-shirt drive, he was one of the first people there. We talked a bit, and I explained to him how I felt. He assured me that he didn't mean any harm and that he would try to be more supportive. I was ok with that.

I wanted him to tell me I was beautiful when I didn't have a strand of hair or rub my back and tell me everything was going to be ok even if it wasn't.

After the fish fry, he asked me if he could tell me something and made me promise not to be mad. I promised. That's when he told me he had been seeing someone else. I thought it was kind of funny because there was no way that he could have possibly believed that I thought he wasn't. We weren't doing anything together, and we didn't see each other. He would call occasionally and tell me sweet nothings, but it didn't go anywhere, and I didn't have any expectations on it doing so. I guess it was just the mature thing for him to do, considering what was on my plate.

That night, I sat in his car with him and cried for so long, my mom fell asleep in the car behind us, while waiting for me. I didn't cry because it was over, I didn't cry because he was seeing someone else, I didn't cry for any other reason, but the fact that I was engaged to this man and with him for damn near six years, and now when I needed him the most, he couldn't fully be there the way I needed him to be. I wanted him to be there to hold and cater to me. I wanted him to tell me I was beautiful when I didn't have a strand of hair or rub my back and tell me everything was going to be ok even if it wasn't. Part of the conversation we had led me to believe that he wanted to continue the conversation from inside, but we didn't. He sat there and I poured my heart out in tears as I cried. We hardly said any words. I just cried. I felt like a part of him may have been heartbroken for me.

You must be careful about what you ask for. Things had gotten so bad with us at some point in our relationship; I guess he had gotten comfortable. I was in the house alone all the time. I had become so lonely that I wanted to be sick, just so he could be a little more attentive to me. I got way more than what I bargained for. People have lied to me, and I have been betrayed. But I had never felt this type of pain before. I had never been this hurt. I felt like I couldn't breathe.

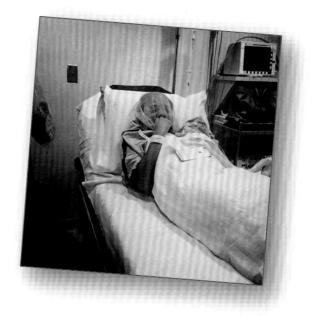

It was a long ride home as I replayed what he said over and over in my head. I had to let go of what was already gone for the sake of my sanity and health; and had to remind myself of how strong I was. I decided to turn my pain into fuel to feed my strength. I needed to be as healthy as possible mentally, physically, and emotionally. Moving forward, he was as supportive as he could be respectfully. During that time, he became one of my best friends. I was happy that we were able to remain friends.

Even though I hated going to Einstein to have my exams done, I chose my family doctor based on her experience and reviews. Had I known that if something were to happen, I would have to deal with this hospital, I probably would have chosen another family doctor. Traveling to Broad and Olney was a headache. It was one of the most congested bus depots here in the city. Parking is always a B****, not to mention needing change to park, and finding someone to give you some. I had to figure out something else when it came to this place.

That's why choosing a location to be treated was essential. I had to figure out what factors would be relevant to me; and that was location and convenience. I wanted a prime location close to work and home. I needed to be able to get to my appointments that were early morning, after work, or last-minute appointments. I also wanted to be able to get to my appointments if it was inclement weather. I needed doctors with full availability, so I could move my dates and times that best fit my schedule with minimal to no inconvenience.

I chose to continue seeing Dr. Zimmerman at The Fox Chase Cancer Center. I'm not even going to sit here and lie to try to convince anyone that I did all this homework and extensively researched my doctors because I didn't. When the hospital scheduled me with a doctor is when I figured out who I would be seeing, and then I googled them. If I was comfortable with what I read, then we moved forward. However, if I was unsatisfied, then I rescheduled with someone else. I looked him up and checked his experience practicing Oncology. After all, I was hiring him for an important job. I needed him to help me save my life.

He was a shorter Caucasian man, maybe around his late 30's to early 40's. He was cute too. His energy was high, and he seemed to be a sincere, respectful man. He was polite and shared more of a personal relationship with his patients, or maybe it was just my family and me. I believed he had my best interest. His bedside manner was on point. He went with the flow of things. Whatever I was on, he was on. If I was serious, he was too. If I made light of a situation, he did the same. Unless it was something very serious. When picking a doctor, it is important to like and care for them because you are in better spirits when seeing them and you are comfortable discussing your issues with them. I looked forward to seeing Dr. Zimmerman. That was a good sign.

During the conversation, I learned that sometimes, the chemotherapy treatment can cause sterilization. As a result, my ovaries had to be suppressed, so they didn't produce any hormones (i.e. estrogen or progesterone) which could potentially feed my cancer and cause it to progress. It also provided shelter from the harm of the chemotherapy.

He offered me the opportunity to see a fertility doctor to freeze my eggs. Oocyte Cryopreservation is the technical term for the method of freezing eggs. I needed to start treatment immediately after completing the procedure if I opted to do the procedure.

I selected the Abington Hospital Fertility Clinic. During my initial visit, the office seemed neat and welcoming. There were plenty of pictures of babies and things that transpire in your body during the process. My mother and I sat there and talked for a long while about how we thought things would go and the cost and the procedure itself. It bothered me so much; my stomach was hurting, thinking about what the price of this would be.

The assistant was patient and polite as she showed me to my designated room. The doctor asked me an ample amount of questions regarding previous pregnancies and sexual partners, etc. All was well as my mom sat in the room, paying close attention, making sure not to miss anything important. Then he asked, "have you ever had any sexually transmitted diseases?"

I can't explain the look on my face in words knowing I had to admit to having a venereal disease. This would have been okay, but not in front of my mom.

"Yes," I responded.
Then he asked, "Which ones?"

I responded, "Chlamydia and Gonorrhea," to which my mother immediately asked.
"Well, who the hell gave you a venereal disease?"

She was furious! I ignored her and pretended to be waiting for the doctor to ask me something else. The next question seemed to be taking FOREVER! "God, please hurry up and have him ask this next question," I said to myself. When I turned to my left, she was sitting there looking with the (I'm waiting) look. So, I told her who and she was hot! It's safe to say she doesn't like him anymore even though it was years ago. I guess because it was new to her. By that time, I was long over it.

Next, we discussed the finances, which was about $15,000/$25,000 dollars! That price included visits, egg retrieval, and medication. There was also a $500 fee annually, for the storage of the eggs.

"OMG! I'll never be able to afford this!" I told myself I wasn't going to cry, but I soon felt the tears trickle down my cheeks. I didn't know if I wanted to have kids, but the thought of not being able to have the option was very catastrophic.

... my mother immediately asked. "Well, who the hell gave you a venereal disease?"

After considering my age and diagnosis, they were waiving all the fees. I would only be responsible for the storage charges yearly. My mom and I cried. I couldn't have been more grateful. That was the first time I'd ever cried tears of joy. The blessings continuously fell upon me. That was something else I could take off my plate.

The procedure was a little more complicated than I expected. After a few days, I received a big box in the mail. When I opened it, it was all types of medical supplies; alcohol pads, syringes, medicine, a box to discard the used needles, etc.

For three weeks, I had to inject myself daily with a syringe filled with the fertility hormone, progesterone, used to stimulate ovulation. I remember the first day counting to ten… 1, 2, 3, 4, 5 before I could stick myself with the needle and then having to count again because I just couldn't bring myself to do it.

So, I went to my next option. "Mom, help me with this needle. I can't do it." "Neeky," she said, "how am I supposed to help you? You know you have a weak stomach."

So, I counted again. I may have counted about seven times before I stuck myself. To my

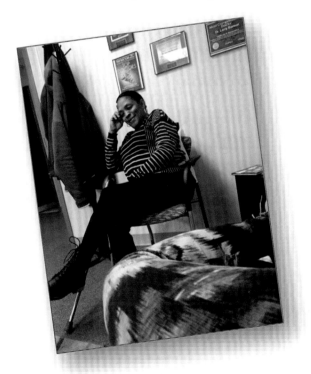

surprise, it was just a small pinch, and it was over. The anticipation of administering the medication was more traumatic than the actual needle. Over time, I got used to it, but the anxiety about sticking myself never got any better. I still had to count every day.

About a week after starting the medication, the pain started. The pain in my back was from ovulating. My ovaries were working overtime, and I felt every bit of it. It had me questioning the whole thing. "Am I going to even want to have a baby after feeling the pain just to produce some eggs?" I take my hat off to all mothers; I applaud the mothers who give birth with no epidural. They are something like supernatural.

Motrin nor Ibuprofen could provide any relief. I was in so much pain, I needed some pressure applied to that area. Luckily for me, a friend of mine was always available to massage my back. He regularly rubbed my back where the pain was. I'm so grateful for him. He was there to help me through the whole thing. Don't worry about my happy ending. Ha ha!

Three weeks later, the day of retrieval. I sat in the examination chair that reclined and had a footrest; the type women sit in when they see the Gynecologist.

The doctor explained to me the whole process: "I will insert a needle with a catheter attached to it, inside your vagina. Then, with light suction, I will remove each grape-like egg from your ovaries. They will then be placed in sterile test tubes and labeled with your name and identification number. An Embryologist will handle them from there. You only require slight anesthesia, so you should be alert 15-20 minutes after the procedure is complete. There is no downtime afterward so that you can continue with your day as you wish. But everyone is different; you may need to rest. There may be some slight bleeding, but don't be alarmed that is completely normal."

"Am I going to even want to have a baby after feeling the pain just to produce some eggs?"

He reclined my chair and administered the anesthesia. I fell completely asleep because I don't remember a thing. When I regained consciousness, I thought I was in the room alone. However, my family was right there, and I felt fine. The doctor came in to make sure I was ok, and I was free to go.

Ultimately there were 10 eggs retrieved and 5 of them were mature enough to store. Following egg retrieval, my ovaries were suppressed.

The medication Zolodex is given once every 28 days. Each time the side of my stomach alternates. The process consists of two steps. First using one syringe of Lidocaine to numb the site. After allowing that some time to reach its full potential strength the medication is administered with another needle. Finally, the site is cleaned and bandaged.

Tina was the nurse who would be administering my shot. She explained the procedure, "I'm going to numb the area with the Lidocaine. It will sting a bit, and then we will let it sit for a while. When I come back, I will administer the shot, and you won't feel a thing." She used an alcohol pad to sterilize the site. Next, she administered the Lidocaine, which did sting a bit, but nothing I couldn't handle. She gave it 15 minutes to get to its full strength. I sat there looking through magazines and stealing pages of recipes I wanted to try.

When she came back, she tested the site to see if it was numb. It wasn't numb because I could feel the pricking she was doing. (Which was taking the edge of the alcohol pad package and pressing it against the site). She set the timer and returned in 10 minutes. I still didn't believe it was numb enough. Then, she said, "if we wait too long, it will stop working altogether." I thought about it. "If this stops working, this is going to hurt seriously." So, I allowed her to proceed.

She cleaned the area off a second time with another alcohol pad. She opened the package that concealed the needle, and I could have passed out at the size of it. I couldn't understand what could cause that needle to be that big. It was the biggest needle I had ever seen in my life.

"What's in that needle?" I asked.
"Oh, the medication is actually in pellet form."
She put it against my skin and pushed the top down, which disbursed a pellet into my stomach.
"AHHH!" I screamed in agony.

I could see the look of concern in Tina's face as she apologized profusely. I could tell it was sincere. But I couldn't care less. That hurt like hell! It felt exactly like what it was, a big behind needle going into my stomach. It only hurt for a few moments. But I would have instead not felt it at all. On everything I loved, she would never touch me again. Let alone give me a needle.

Directly before starting treatment, I had to have an Echocardiogram to make sure my heart was strong enough to withstand it. Trying to schedule my Echocardiogram was just as gruesome as the other scans at Einstein. After multiple calls, holding, and being transferred, I was finally scheduled, but with a date three months out. Which would mean my treatment would be delayed even further. It was terribly upsetting that they had no concern for the urgency of my health condition. After going back and forth and speaking with multiple supervisors, managers, and schedulers, would you believe I still had the same appointment? Finally, I expressed my issue with my oncologist. He called Einstein himself and got me an appointment for later that week so that I could start my treatment as soon as possible.

My Echocardiogram's duration was about 45 minutes. The course of action was like my biopsy ultrasound, except for the biopsy part. The sono-tech used a transducer and applied jelly to it. Then, put it against my skin right above my heart. The sensor later recorded the soundwave echoes that my heart produced. Then, they were interchanged into moving figures on a computer screen.

TREATMENT PLAN

I always thought that when a treatment plan was selected for a patient, it's original to the individual. However, I learned that treatment plans are based on the diagnosis. Everyone with that specific diagnosis will most likely have the same treatment plan options. Either you need surgery, radiation, or chemotherapy or you don't. One may require a Lumpectomy, a complete or Bilateral Mastectomy.

In my case, I needed surgery. But the best surgery and treatment plan still had to be determined. Dr. Zimmerman previously explained that surgery would be after six weeks of an aggressive chemotherapy treatment that would shrink the tumor and would take place before maintenance treatments. My life would be consumed with countless appointments, scans, treatments, surgeries, checkups, etc. for the next year and maybe even longer. I needed to see the breast surgeon, Dr. Li, and plastic reconstruction surgeon, Dr. Hamilton.

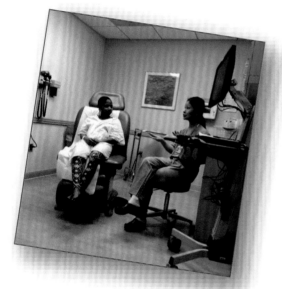

I did the same research ritual. GOOGLE! I looked at Dr. Hamilton's work, and I was satisfied with what I saw. During my appointment, he explained my options of ways to remove the tumors and reconstruction in further detail. He also had a few sample implants for me to check out.

A Lumpectomy would have been the first option, but it was out of the question because I had too many significant sized tumors. That procedure would more than likely leave my affected breast deformed. So, a complete or Bilateral Mastectomy of the right breast would be the next option to consider. After either Mastectomy, the reconstruction would be a lengthy process, if I decided to get implants. But, if I got a flap tram, the reconstruction would be immediately after.

The implants consisted of placing an expander under the tissue. Expanders are balloon-like except that they have a port on them, where more fluid is added to increase the size while under the skin. They are placed under the breastbone, and they stretch the surface enough for the placement of the desired implant dimensions. This procedure usually takes 6-8 weeks before you can have the implants placed. There is minimal scarring and downtime to recover.

I've heard many horror stories about implants. The one that perturbed me the most was that they may burst. I can't begin to imagine how the hell they would correct such a thing. "Would I want to go through another procedure to correct something out of my control?" I asked myself. That was concerning enough for me to cross implants off my list of prospects immediately.

A flap tram is a procedure of taking some of the muscle, blood vessels, and fat from the lower part of the stomach near the bikini line. These contents are then molded into a breast shape and used in place of what would be an implant. Then, skin is taken from what becomes available from the stomach to replace the nipples. During this process, the belly button is typically removed, repositioned, and returned.

Another option was no reconstruction at all. That would mean I would be entirely flat-chested on each side operated on without nipples, depending on if it was a complete or Bilateral Mastectomy. They would stitch me up directly afterward. Radiation wouldn't be required for the total Mastectomy. But it would still be necessary for the bilateral. For me, this was not even an option. Being 30 and single, I wanted to look and feel as much like a normal 30-year-old as possible.

I would be losing the opportunity to breastfeed, which is a significant factor in motherhood.

On the other hand, when considering a double Mastectomy, I thought this to be the best option for me. It took inhibitory measures and didn't require any radiation. It consisted of eradicating all the breast tissue, even the tissue that wasn't influenced. It still followed six aggressive treatments. Then, finally, numerous maintenance treatments. After crossing the other reconstruction options off my list, I was left with the flap tram.

Sadly, this would leave the most scarring and would require the most downtime. There would be a massive scar at my hips, which would be across from one side to the other. The best part of this procedure was that I would have a flat stomach afterward. The worst part was that I would be losing the opportunity to ever breastfeed, which is a significant factor in motherhood. So, I viewed it as a tummy tuck and breast lift. That made the procedure a bit more intriguing. After selecting the double Mastectomy with a flap tram, I was able to move on to the next step.

A port-a-cath is the proper name for the device, also known as a port. It is a temporary tube placed in a vein near the heart used to collect blood samples, assisting with administering medication and dialysis, i.e., intravenous fluids, blood transfusions, chemotherapy, and other drugs. It makes connecting an IV less complicated and cuts downtime with needles and accessing veins.

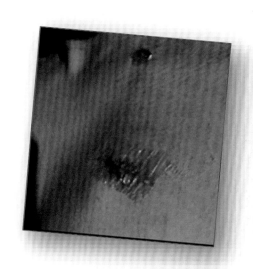

I had the port placed on the opposite side of the affected side. So, for me, it was placed on the left side,

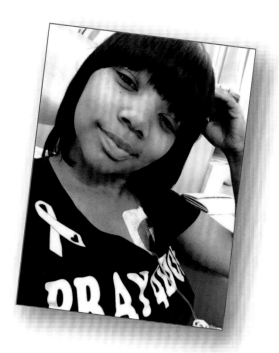

under the skin on my chest. The anesthesia was like the sedation for egg retrieval. After the procedure, I wasn't in any pain. I just had a little discomfort and I could see my skin raised where the port was.

Preparing for my chemotherapy was mental for me. After hearing so many rumors about chemo, I just knew my skin was about to melt off and be used as gasoline to fuel cars. So, I decided not to do much reading about cancer, the medication, and symptoms. I wanted to have my own experiences, rather than imagine the ones of

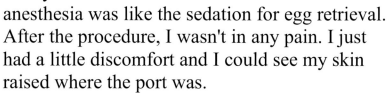

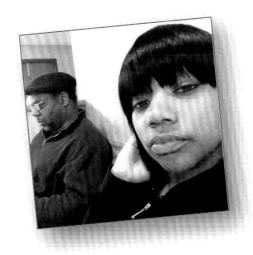

others. My treatment started immediately after having my eggs retrieved and port placed, as my doctor stated it would.

I was required to do six rounds of aggressive treatment. They were once every three weeks to allow time for my body to repair itself before the next round. The medications I would be taking were Benadryl, Neoadjuvant, Carboplatin, Herceptin, Perjecta, and Docetaxel.

On the day of my first treatment, I walked into the Fox Chase Cancer Center, ready for war. Of course, I had my mom, dad, and brother with me.

My dad's name is Kevin. We have more of a friendship bond. He is more laid back and chill, almost opposite of my mom. No shade, but he's the more relaxed parent. The parent you don't have shame to tell anything to. I used to be so worried about people not liking me. He made me feel better about it because he doesn't care about what most people think about him.

He said, "Everybody ain't going to like you; that's life." From that day forward, I handled my emotions about the way people think of me differently. IDGAF!

My brother, Devin, was also there. He's my little big brother. I used to beat him up all the time, until one day I didn't win. We are just shy of 2 years apart.

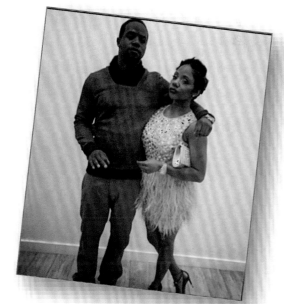

I went to the receptionist's desk and gave my name and date of birth. After they verified everything with the wristband, they put it around my wrist. We sat in the waiting room until my name was called.

When I heard my name, I went to get my complete blood count. They were checking my red and white cells as well as the platelets. My counts had to be sufficient to be treated.

The nurse sterilized the area where my port was. She used a small needle and accessed it. Then, she inserted a needle connected to a short IV line in the bubble of the port and I felt a sharp pain. Next, she flushed it with saline to make sure the line is clear and working smoothly. Instantly, there was a nasty taste that filled my mouth and seemed to come out of my nose. It tasted like metal. The blood flowed into about five tubes quickly. Lastly, she flushed it, and again the same taste filled my mouth and nose. The nurse covered my port with a plastic tape dressing called Tegaderm, and I went back to the waiting room with my family.

Instantly, there was a nasty taste that filled my mouth and seemed to come out of my nose. It tasted like metal.

After sitting there for about 45 minutes, I got up to see how much longer the wait would be; that's when I learned I was in the wrong place. Apparently, I needed to see my oncologist after having my blood work completed. I was pissed because I felt that someone should have told me what to do since this was my first time doing this. I was directed to where I would see my oncologist, Dr. Zimmerman.

During my appointment, he answered my questions and explained my next steps and what to expect. He also let me know that the first few treatments would be quite lengthy, due to a grace period between medications. There is a slower drip enforced for safety precautions and checks for unwanted side effects from the medicines.

After my visit, I returned to the reception desk again — this time, I received a pager. I sat in the waiting room and talked to my family. Surprisingly, I wasn't scared. I was just ready to get it over with at this point. I sat there about a half-hour or forty-five minutes before my pager went off.

Because there were only 1-2 guests permitted in the infusion room at a time with each patient, my mother came in with me first. In the infusion room, there were a bunch of recliners with pillows lined up with one or two chairs alongside them and a personal TV. Each chair had a number beginning at one and going all the way up to about 40. There was a nursing station in the middle of the floor occupied by plenty of nurses and assistants.

She replied, "don't let your mind play tricks on you..."

I went into the triage first where I had my blood pressure and weight taken. The tech asked me a whole bunch of questions I felt were unnecessary, but it was protocol, I guess! I was uninterested until she asked, "Do you want a warm blanket?" Throughout the whole time I received treatment, I would look forward to those warm blankets.

I was taken to chair six and introduced to the nurse who would be treating me. I sat down, and they flushed my port and connected it to the infusion pump. I had the same after taste with the flush. At this point, the flush had been the worst part. The nurse offered us coffee, donuts, juice, or water and then went to fetch our desires. While I was waiting for her to return, I felt the meds kicking in. All the symptoms I heard about were hitting me at once. I was starting to feel sick, light-headed, and I began to be nauseous.

When my nurse returned, I informed her of the symptoms I was experiencing. I was concerned because I didn't believe how fast the symptoms were hitting me. I wanted to make sure it was typical. She replied, "don't let your mind play tricks on you. I've only connected you to the machine. Your medication is still in the pharmacy. Just relax, I promise it's not as bad as you probably think."

It was all in my head. I wasn't experiencing any symptoms. The mind can cause paranoia, confusion, anxiety, and for sure, hallucination. I watched some tv shows as my family rotated sitting with me. I remember looking at the machine drip. It seemed to take forever. By the time it was over, I was beat. I mean it literally, drained of every ounce of my energy. I felt fine besides that.

My nurse did my final flush, and that same nasty taste from the saline followed. This time I complained, the nurse suggested I chew gum or eat a mint during the flush. She said that should help with the after taste. She removed the port access and applied a bandage. Just like that I was done. If it was going to be this easy, "I got this!" I thought. I was in for a rude awakening; this was only a taste of what I had to endure.

My initial treatment lasted for about 8 hours. During that time, I urinated an uncountable amount of times. I tried to hold my urine until the end of my treatment. But I just couldn't. I was receiving medication in fluid form; my bladder was filling swiftly. I hated that I had to take the IV pump with me each time. It was just a hassle. I had to unplug it and drag it to the bathroom. Then, pull it all the way back.

Chemotherapy attacks your white blood cells. As a result, to protect yourself you must stay out of crowded places and wear a face mask to protect yourself from germs and parasites. Because my immune system was suppressed, my body wouldn't be able to fight off infections; any infection could possibly kill me. In the beginning, it can be challenging because everyone treats you as if you have the plague. I remember being out and feeling embarrassed because people would be staring at me. My mom witnessed it and asked this lady "haven't you ever taught your kids about staring?" Even though I am grown, she still takes up for me. I felt like a kid again. In my head I was saying, "Yeah, tell her mom!"

After each aggressive treatment I had to have a bone marrow stimulant. Nuelasta is an on-body injector that helps make white blood cells. It would be taped to the back of my arm and if it's applied correctly it beeps once and the indicator flashes a green light. After having my injector placed for 22 hours, I took Claritin with hopes of not withstanding the main symptom, bone pain. Gratefully, I never experienced that.

At the 24th hour the injector sounds a series of beeps before the medication is administered.

The next three weeks flew by. I was astounded that I had not witnessed any symptoms from the medication. I wasn't complaining either. Just happy to be in better spirits than I expected. Before I knew it, it was time for treatment again.

The second treatment was pretty much the same. I tried to eat a mint during my flush, but I got no relief. The pain of the port access and the duration of the treatment remained the same. I saw Dr. Zimmerman, regularly for mostly short visits between treatments. He checked to make sure I felt ok and didn't have any questions or concerns.

MAINTAINING MY REGULAR ROUTINE

I continued to work through my treatment. Part of the reason is because most people seem to learn of their diagnosis of cancer and stop living. They succumb to the disease without even trying to fight. So, because I was lucky enough to have the strength to operate normally, I would do so.

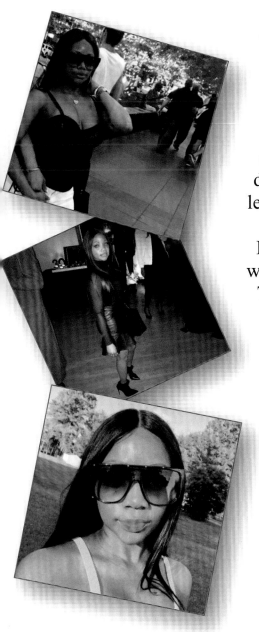

My mom was upset because I continued to work. However, it gave me a purpose and kept me motivated. Working and keeping my routine as close as it was before I was diagnosed, kept me levelheaded.

I worked out a routine with my coworker, Tiffany. At the beginning of the week, I would cover the bulk of the work; that's when I had the most energy. Towards the end of the week, she would cover the job because I would be physically drained from my treatment. I guess by now you can see, I don't like to call out of work either.

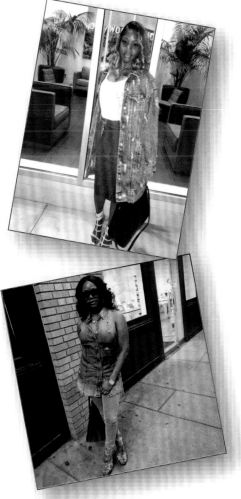

In addition to going to work, I got up and went to the mall, to dinner, to happy hour, and I even went on a few dates. Being as though I was single, there was no need not to share all this good loving I still had to offer. Even though I was staying home, I still had bills. I chose to fight and live my life versus fight lying down. With that attitude, I was able to fight my battle graciously. I stayed in the house and did DIY projects; I made wigs and got good over time, reupholstered furniture, and I played in my makeup. I didn't become a certified MUA, but I did do a damn good job concealing my imperfections due to the chemotherapy.

SYMPTOMS

The third treatment was about the same, except the length of the treatment. Each time they were a bit shorter. I was down to about 5 hours. Yet, following this treatment, I started to experience some of the common side effects.

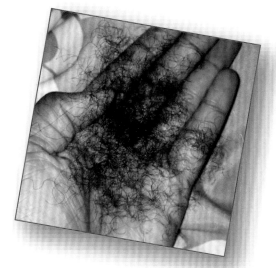

I secretly wished and prayed that I would be the first person who didn't experience hair loss during this treatment. My scalp began to get sore, and small amounts of my hair started to fall out. Although I knew my hair would fall out, I didn't know my scalp would be sore. I decided before I started being treated that when my hair began to fall out, I would cut it. It seemed that it would be so discouraging to watch my hair fall out. So, I would beat the disease at its own game and cut my hair myself.

ℛ

I secretly wished and prayed that I would be the first person who didn't experience hair loss during this treatment.

ℛ

One day, while in the shower, I noticed the amount of hair I was losing was greater than before. I got out of the shower and dried off. I had purposely been avoiding the mirror when my hair wasn't covered. I looked at myself and my hair in the mirror for the first time in a long time. I saw how much thinner it was. That's when I noticed that most of my eyebrows and lashes were also gone. When I previously thought of losing my hair, I only thought about the hair on

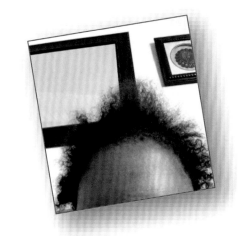

my head. I never considered that I would lose my eyebrows and lashes and hair on my private area as well. I preferred to keep my private sector clean anyway, so that wasn't an issue, but losing my eyebrows and lashes only made me feel uglier. I lost so many things I never even thought about being grateful for.

I went to get my scissors and came back to the bathroom. I put a towel on the floor and closed the door. In no particular style, I cut what hair remained on my head. I was only able to cut it to a specific length safely using the scissors. So, then I got my clippers and neatly shaved my head. I didn't have an audience. I didn't even care for one. I didn't need anyone crying and causing me to cry. Cutting my hair was genuinely liberating. My bald head didn't look that bad on me either.

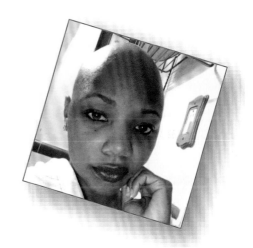

I wanted to play around and see how I looked "**bald and glammed**". I grabbed some lip liner, lipstick, and my favorite brow pencil. After applying all, I was amazed at how good "bald and glammed" looked on me. I went downstairs. My mom was on the couch. She tried not to seem shocked, but of course, she was.

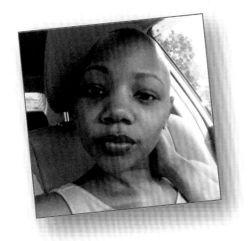

"You actually look cute with a bald head. Mostly because it's small and not funny shaped," I heard her say while on my way to the kitchen. She believed that it complimented me more than anything. My grandmom shaping my head when I was a baby, finally served its purpose.

The magnitude of encouragement and compliments I received after revealing my bald head encouraged me, even after someone shared my picture in the *Spice Gang* group on Facebook. I read all the cruel jokes about my looks and I still kept my head up. I was surprised how much more comfortable I felt after I shared with everyone.

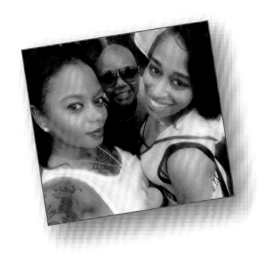

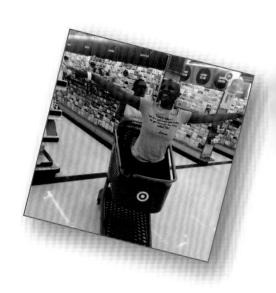

I told myself I would never come outside with my bald head, but after some time, I grew comfortable enough with "the temporary new me" to do so. Eventually, I became so confident that I didn't try to cover it, from a few strands to peach fuzz that grew into a small afro, I walked around freely. The most important thing I possessed during the entire ordeal was confidence. My hair didn't define me. My appearance on the outside may have been ugly to me, but it wasn't to others. If someone did think I was ugly, that was a major "F" for them.

My fingertips were beginning to be sore and tingly, and my nails seemed to be thinning. The tingling was a symptom of Neuropathy. Neuropathy can be numbness or weakness, and sometimes pain in the feet and/or hands, and if it's caught soon enough it is reversible. I was only suffering from minimum nausea at this point.

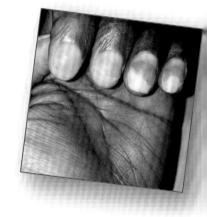

❧

The most important thing I possessed during the entire ordeal was confidence.

❧

So far, the worst part of this were my taste buds because they were altered. It brings tears to my eyes just to think about it. It's the hardest thing trying to describe the taste. An example is to imagine drinking a glass of water, and it tasted like sucking on rusty costume jewelry. I once enjoyed spicy food, but now eating spicy food literally felt like fire dancing on my tongue. Food that was seasoned perfectly would always seem to need more seasoning; only to add more seasoning for it to taste even worse. I started drinking Ensures to make sure I got some nutrients because my appetite was obsolete.

On the better side of things, my taste buds began to revert about 2 or 3 days before my next treatment. After not having an appetite for weeks, BABY! I binged. I ate everything I craved for the past three weeks. I was losing weight by not eating well and lacking proper nutrients. But, I would gain all of it back within those few days that my taste buds were regressing. Throughout this time, my weight fluctuated between 110-114lbs.

Rasul, a friend of mine came to see me one day, he had so many Ensures; it had to be damn near 100 bottles. I had to find somewhere to store them all. He bought chocolate, strawberry, and dark chocolate. I was so grateful. After a while, those flavors got boring. That's when I found butter pecan. OMG! My favorite of all. I couldn't find them in stores, so I had to purchase them online at Amazon.

My fourth treatment was my most brief treatment, but the symptoms only intensified and lasted longer each time. At this point, my nails were painful and separating from my nail bed. My skin was dark and very sore at the front and inner sides of my knees between my legs.

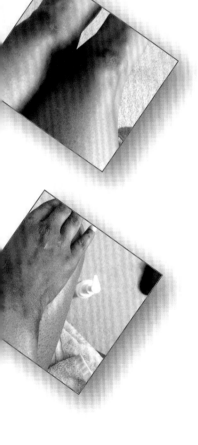

My skin was so dry it began peeling at my feet and hands. The peeling was so severe it felt hot. Dr. Zimmerman advocated for Udderly Smooth cream. It wasn't strong enough for the task. I desired a stronger cream with a steroid additive called Cutivate Ointment. I already had Eczema, so that was something that I had utilized prior to chemotherapy. He wrote me a prescription for the cream.

Although I liked the ointment better, I was relieved. Anything was better than that over-the-counter bull crap he suggested the first time. That stuff was a joke!

I wasn't going to keep attempting to eat regular food without being able to enjoy it. My mom came up with an experiment. She'd make something I had never had before. I didn't have any expectations of how it should taste. So, I couldn't be disappointed.

She made chicken gizzard soup with livers, carrots, and potatoes. It may sound nasty but, it was the best thing I had to eat in months. I enjoyed every drop of it. I probably wouldn't eat it today though. It still didn't help with my appetite. I didn't have the slightest urge to eat. I was becoming dehydrated, my lips were white, cracking, and sometimes even bleeding. I used Chapstick and Blistex to moisturize them. Unfortunately, that started to burn because the skin at the corner of my mouth cracked. That was irritating but only painful when I tried to put something on it, or something got in it.

My tongue was white. I was always in the mirror, trying to scrape whatever it was off. It was disgusting. I would be gagging the entire time. I had no idea what it was. So, I Googled it like I did everything else. I'm sure you can probably relate. Google said it was oral thrush and oral Lichen Planus. Both of those things had to do with a weakened immune system and dehydration. It also mentioned that it could be the early stages of cancer and is caused by antibiotics and a bunch of other things. Dr. Zimmerman assured me that it was normal and would clear up on its own, and it did.

By my fifth treatment, the medicine had finally taken over my body completely.

It was pitiful, and it indeed lowered my spirits.

By my fifth treatment, the medicine had finally taken over my body completely. My fingernails were entirely off, and my fingertips were sore to the touch. Both of my big toenails had totally detached and had fallen off. It was quite upsetting for me because I am very particular about my feet and toenails. Summer was approaching, and I loved wearing my feet out. Now I wasn't going to be able to. It was pitiful, and it indeed lowered my spirits.

I was constantly throwing up. But, because I was hardly eating or drinking, there was merely any contents in my stomach. I was dry heaving and gagging. It was so frustrating. The Zofran (anti-nausea medicine) wasn't working. I tried to smoke weed and I didn't get any relief, contrary to many people's beliefs.

My sleep regimen was so poor. I was hardly sleeping even after trying several different sleep aides. Though I was physically, mentally, and emotionally exhausted, I still couldn't fall asleep. I was suffering from the worst case of insomnia that I had ever observed. I would lie in bed for hours before I would start to cry from being so frustrated. I don't praise this, but I started to try things off the street to help me sleep. I tried to smoke weed again. That worked slightly; it only cut the time that it took me to fall asleep. I would still toss and turn for long periods. Then, I tried "lean", which is a cough syrup that contains Promethazine. That helped a bit, but not like I needed. Dr. Zimmerman prescribed me a few medications for sleep; each one hardly helped. One of them was Nortriptyline. I feared that because I remember taking one of my mom's years prior, and I slept for two days.

Why did you choose me to fight this battle?

Why do you think I'm this strong?

What do you want me to learn?

What did I do wrong to deserve this?"

Then, I bought a Xanax 10mg off the street. I cut it in half, and it gave me the results I wished for. I fell asleep quickly and slept all night. However, when I woke up, I hadn't slept the medicine off, and I was drowsy all day. I told Dr. Zimmerman about it, and he prescribed me a 5mg Xanax. I cut that in half, and that was perfect. I was sleeping 7-8 hours and waking up rejuvenated.

I was also suffering from diarrhea, which made my anus raw and painful. At the same time, I was constipated. I'm guessing just by explaining that you can understand the level of annoyance I had, suffering from both constipation and diarrhea at the same damn time. I know it sounds unbelievable, but that's really a "thing".

I often cried to myself because I wanted to seem strong for my family. I didn't want to agonize them any further. I didn't want them to know that I couldn't take the symptoms from the medication any longer. The medicine was making me sicker than the cancer itself. I wanted to cease the treatment and accept whatever my fate would be. I wanted to feel better. I wanted my regular life back. I was defeated; I gave up.

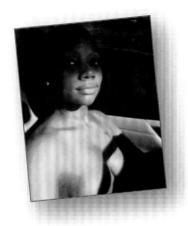

I questioned God at this time:
Why did you choose me to fight this battle?
Why do you think I'm this strong?
What do you want me to learn?
What did I do wrong to deserve this?

I wanted him to reveal whatever I was supposed to learn from this experience, and I wanted to be clear on what my lesson was so I would never have to go through this again. My sixth treatment was a piece of cake. It lasted for 2 hours. I was invited to ring the bell. To ring the bell signifies that you have completed all your treatments. Being as though I still had to have surgery, and countless maintenance treatments, I declined.

By this time, I was suffering from a new symptom - hot flashes. My chemically induced menopause caused them. Now, I understood my mom's "private summers". When I had a hot flash, my body seemed to be overheating. My skin would become moist just moments before the sweat poured out of my glands. I was so ashamed and embarrassed. There was nothing I could do to conceal or hide it.

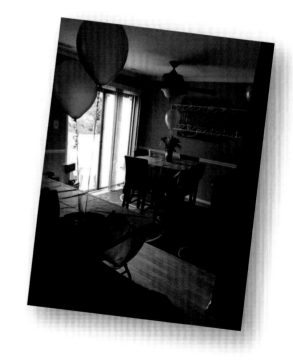

Although I chose not to ring the bell, my friend Dior decided to throw me a "halfway there" cookout at her home. An hour withered away while we were trying to figure out why the grill wouldn't ignite. We finally figured out that we didn't have any gas in the tank. It was the first cookout of the season, and the grill hadn't been used since the year prior, so it was understandable. We searched diligently for a place to fill our propane tank on a late Sunday evening.

We ate and played games. We told our craziest stories about when we were in relationships. That was my favorite part. My friend Bah may have had the most insane stories out of all of us. Most of all we enjoyed each other. Even though some of my friends didn't know each other, they all blended well. It was all love, and I had a great time.

THE
TEA
IS
HOT!

Shortly after completing my aggressive treatments, I was scrolling on Instagram. Social media is a vault of hidden and undiscovered information; that is until it's discovered. Looking over and comparing pictures and videos of the lives of the people you follow is sometimes revealing. Today, the tea spilled, and it was hot!

I saw a few people that I knew attending a baby shower. I didn't pay it any attention at first. But when I paid closer attention, I noticed that all the people had something in common, beyond being at the same shower. They were all the family of my most recent ex-boyfriend, Hass. The one I mentioned before. Yes, him!

I figured I'd do a little investigating and digging. I started looking through the posts of his friends and family on Instagram and Facebook. After reviewing everything, I only had circumstantial evidence. I had watched enough episodes of Law and Order to know I needed something to stick. I couldn't prosecute him with these charges.

I thought back to the time around my fish fry. The timing seemed to add up. Is that why he told me he was seeing someone else?

Today, the tea spilled, and it was hot!

I called my friends and then sent them the evidence (screenshots). I said, "Y'all, I think Hass is having a baby." They all assured me that he would have told me if that was the case. Shucks, I thought he would have told me too. After all, we were friends. I couldn't confirm anything online. So, I broke down and called and asked him. He confirmed that he was having his first baby.

"Well, why didn't you tell me?" I asked.
He replied, "I thought you knew."

However, I believe he probably didn't want to deliver news like that to me at such a trying time in my life. Although people expected me to be upset and hurt, that wasn't the case. When I decided to let go of him, I let go of those feelings that would have caused me to be hurt. I saw him as a friend, and I was genuinely happy for him.

LET'S GET BOTCHED

I went through pre-admission testing which included the typical exams to prepare anyone for surgery. I had my blood drawn and an EKG to make sure my heart was operating correctly. A nurse went over my pre-op instructions and preparations. They were to wash the area with Hibiclens twice a day to help sterilize the area. I didn't like the Hibiclens because it didn't lather like ordinary soap. However, I would use it anyway. I was also given a Five Wishes to fill out.

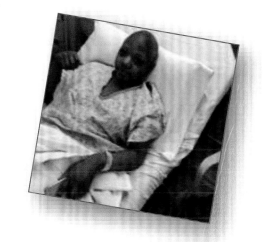

Five Wishes is an advanced directive. The wishes are put in place if you can't make decisions on your own. It covers the kind of medical treatment you want or don't, how comfortable you would like to be, how you want people to treat you, what you would like your loved ones to know, and more. There was even a question about what music I wanted played at my funeral. I always thought about how cool it would be to play "Nann" by Trick Daddy and Trina at my funeral (I love Trina). My mom would probably burn the church down before allowing that though.

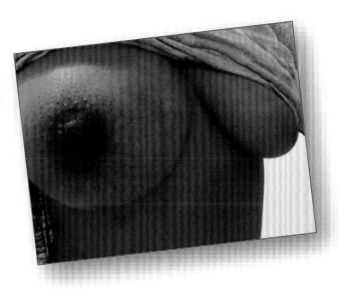

Leading up to my surgery, I had very little anxiety. My biggest fear wasn't the pain. Since I knew I would be asleep, I wasn't worried. I was concerned about how my body would look afterwards with the scars. I didn't know what to expect. I prepared for the worst and prayed for the best.

On the day of my surgery, I arrived at 6 a.m. with my mom, dad, brother, and Aunt. After a short while of sitting in the waiting room, they took me back to the triage to prepare me for surgery. I changed my

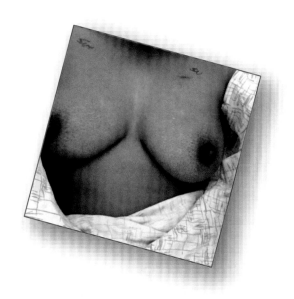

clothes, went to the bathroom to empty my bladder, and provided a urine sample. I had my blood taken and was asked a bunch of pre-surgical questions by a technician, later signing release and consent forms.

It might sound crazy, but I was looking forward to being put to sleep. I figured for the first time in a long time, I would be able to get some good sleep. Dr. Li, my breast surgeon, came in and explained what he would be doing during my procedure and to answer any questions.

Following my breast surgeon, Dr. Hamilton had me stand up and explain what procedure I would be having and he marked the side of my body where he would be operating. My family came in one by one to wish me luck, give me hugs and kisses, and offering prayer. Everyone seemed to be stable until my mom came in.

When she was leaving, I asked, "Mom you're not going to cry, are you?"

She turned around and said, "No," but she had already begun to cry. She's so sensitive. But, I'm her daughter. I can't fathom the amount of pain and worry she felt.

Placing my Intermittent Pneumatic Compression devices on my legs was the final step before surgery. These were cuffs the length of my calves, that filled with air. They were used to prevent blood clots during surgery. The tech gave me something to relax, and that's the last thing I remember.

She turned around and said, "No," but she had already begun to cry.

Seven hours later, I woke up, and I was being wheeled into a room. The first person I remember seeing was P. I remember telling her, "It's gonna be all crop tops and spandex for the summer, this stomach is snatched." I made good on that statement later. When I

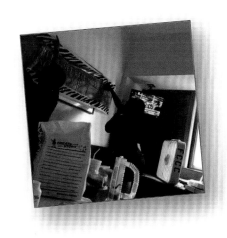

got further into the room, some of my family and friends were there. Some of my other family arrived during my surgery. Two of my friends were decorating my room and hanging my "halfway there" banner from my cookout. There were many flowers, balloons, and cards.

LAWD KNOWS I wasn't prepared for the pain I felt when the meds started to wear off. All the nerves in my breast had been removed, so the pain wasn't coming from there. It was the pain from the incision at my hip. I would describe the pain as an achy soreness compared to working out your abs extremely hard the day before, and I couldn't see the result because, of course, there was swelling. I had plenty of bandages on as well as a bra that looked like a white bulletproof vest. I had a catheter in place to keep my bladder empty during my surgery. Still, the procedure had seemed to have gone well. I had a bit of anxiety when it was time to take my catheter out. I thought it was going to be painful. But it wasn't.

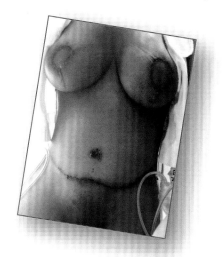

I felt pain whenever I tried to sit up or lay flat. Hell! I felt it every time I moved. So, I tried to stay really, still. But then I had to get up and use the restroom, and the doctors wanted me to walk. I couldn't believe they were neglecting me like this! "I know my rights!" I wanted to say. There was no way they expected me to get up and be moving around so soon after such an invasive surgery, but they insisted.

My nurse Gary was friendly and very attentive. He ended up being classmates with my cousin Asa during nursing school. That didn't help me, though, when he suggested I try to walk to the bathroom. I said, "Nah, I prefer to use the bedpan. I'm not ashamed for you to wipe me either," I was sure he had seen what I had before. I

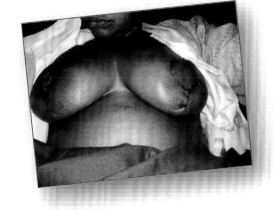

had a fresh shave just in case. Besides that, the bathroom seemed to be 100 miles away. He thought I was hilarious. I was dead serious.

Nonetheless, he made me get up and walk to the bathroom. It wasn't as bad as I anticipated. It was still awful, though, if that makes any sense. I couldn't stand straight up, which made my back hurt. I assumed that I couldn't stand up because of my skin being sewn tighter and not having much elasticity in my abdominal area.

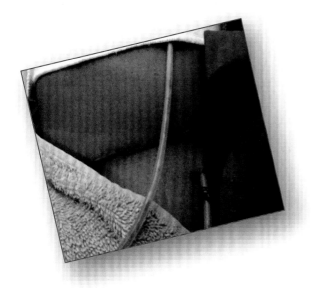

Recovering in the hospital was horrible. After the first day, I had a physical therapist come and assist me with walking down the hall, each day going a little further. I was never able to get proper rest because there were doctors, techs, assistants, and students always in and out of my room. My irritability was through the roof. I think I did an excellent job concealing my attitude, though, because I wanted to tell those students to shove it. They wore me out, asking me the same questions someone else was going to come and ask me again in 5 minutes. I think that should be an option. Not that I don't want people to learn or get experience, but after specific procedures (life-altering), you should have a choice in your own comforts.

When I finally gave my body a look with fewer bandages, I was disgusted to see four clear tubes coming out of my body. There were two on each side. At the end of these tubes were clear balls with a pinkish color fluid in them. They were known as JP drains. They are used to remove the fluid that collects after surgery at the site. They were utterly disgusting.

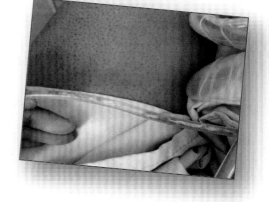

The liquid mixed with blood caused it to be pink. After some time, they started to have long cream strings in them, formed from protein. That made them look even worse. They beat oozing fluid all over the place, on the other hand. I guess! Dr. Hamilton came and spoke with me and told me that the procedure went well. However, it was a bit challenging to complete the tram because he had taken as much tissue out as possible. That explained why I couldn't stand up straight. Therefore, closing the incision at my stomach made it very tight. All that converted in my head was, "Bih, you are snatched, snatched."

Everyone who came to see me brought me food. That was the only pro to recovering in the hospital. I had a variety of every damn thing. The best part of it was that all the food was free. Well, for me, anyway. My favorite was the food from Panera Bread.

ROAD
TO
RECOVERY

I had three surgical bras, which I would rotate wearing. They had to be worn until my follow-up appointment. My breast couldn't be wet for the next three days. Once my drain collection was 1.0-1.5 ounces daily, I could have them removed. I needed to take some time to rest in between being mobile. I scheduled an appointment with physical therapy before being discharged.

During the next couple of weeks, I relaxed in the living room on the couch. My mom was on the other one, and Toby alternated lounges between both of us. I spent most of my time watching Netflix. During this time, I realized there were some pretty good TV shows being televised. I had become so accustomed to watching reality shows I hadn't realized. I watched *Chopped*, *How To Get Away With Murder*, *Wentworth*, *Scandal*, and *Lost*, to name a few. I grew to appreciate real scripted television again and lost all interest in reality TV shows all together.

I had some people stop by and see me while I was sick. My girlfriend Seven, who was pregnant at the time, came over and watched a movie with me. Marcus came and watched a movie with me as well. It may seem minor, but stuff like that sticks with you forever. Especially, since some people I considered friends never even called to check on me, let alone visited. Think about it, when is the last time you had a friend watch a movie with you? I'll wait! Anyway, we watched *The Fault In Our Stars*. Even though it made me cry every time, I loved watching that movie.

It may seem minor, but stuff like that sticks with you forever.

After being cooped up for so long, I decided to take my mom up on an offer to get out. It was an early summer afternoon. The sky was clear, and the sun was shining. I could smell the summer air and see the kids playing football on the lawns across the street. I was so excited to get out. We were going to Home Depot, and I was ecstatic. Luckily, I was proactive and purchased some oversized dresses to slip on after surgery to possibly conceal my bandages. It was smart thinking because now I needed to hide my JP drains as well. I pinned each of my drains to the hem

I'm forever grateful for the sacrifices my friends made during this time.

inside my denim dress with a small safety pin. Afterward, I had two on each side. I was impressed at the excellent job I did concealing them.

I went out with my bald head as usual. It became too hot sometimes to keep it covered up. I strolled around with my mom for a few hours. Unfortunately, my stomach still hadn't stretched enough for me to stand up completely. So, I had to walk around using the walker my aunt gave me so I could slump over a bit. Occasionally my back would ache, and I had to take time to rest on the chair of the walker.

I enjoyed my time out. However, it was a lot on my body too soon. I had to continue to allow my body to rest. I could gradually do things, but to be out and walking throughout such a vast place was just too strenuous. I continued to do more things little by little, pushing myself to do a bit more each time over the next several weeks. I continued to go to my follow-ups until it was time to get the ball rolling once again.

At one of my follow-up appointments with Dr. Hamilton, I discussed my concerns about the cosmetic part of my surgery, and he informed me that revisions are typically not considered within 6 months of initial surgery. So basically, I had to continue to let my body heal before revisiting the conversation about my imperfections. It also set me back with having my nipples formed and tattoo coloring.

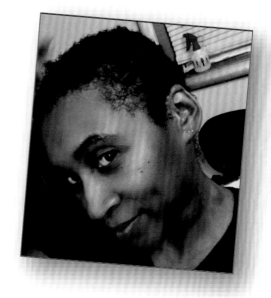

Right before I began my treatments again, my girlfriend Carter cut her hair off in honor of me. It was such a selfless act. I'm forever grateful for the sacrifices my friends made during this time.

BACK

TO

MY

(ALMOST)

REGULARLY

SCHEDULED

PROGRAM

The treatments following my surgery were considered maintenance treatments. Unlike the aggressive treatments, they were very short, and mild enough to allow my hair to start growing back. From the time I came into the treatment room until the time I finished would be about 45 minutes to an hour. As soon as I would get comfortable, it would be time for me to go.

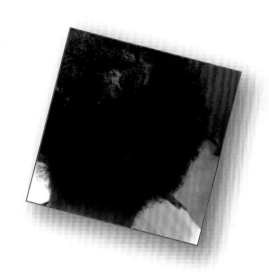

On the weeks when there were holidays is when stuff hit the fan. I can recall becoming so angry from waiting 3 to 4 hours just for treatment. My palms would be sweating, and I would be curving my tongue. I would be livid and ready to cuss people the hell out. Even though my appointment for my Zoladex shot would only be about 30 minutes, sometimes I would be sitting in there 3 to 4 hours as well. Waiting!

I expected to wait a while, but that was just outrageous. One time I was so tired of waiting; I left. I still had my port accessed. When I left, I called the facility and said I had to come back the next day. They went on telling me about protocol, how and what I should have done. I was fed up. "I'll be there in the morning," I said, and ended the call.

When I came back in the morning, I was first. I thought I was slick. I said, "Well, I'll do this every time so I can be in and out. That was until my insurance company got a hold of me. The protocol is that the patient is to be treated the day the port is accessed. You would never understand how petty those insurance companies are until you are sick and need them. They try to skip out on the bill using whatever reason they can find.

You would never understand how petty those insurance companies are until you are sick and need them.

I met plenty of nurses during this whole ordeal, whose names I don't remember. However, there was one whose name I will never forget. Her name was Shelly, and she outweighed them all on so many levels. I always looked forward to seeing her during every visit. I would make sure the other nurses knew she was who I wanted to be my nurse and I would be disappointed when she wasn't there. But, hey, she needed days off too. So many people seemed to not enjoy their job, and it was written all over their faces. It shows in their actions. You can feel it in their energy.

But Shelly, she seemed to like her occupation. She was like a breath of fresh air, always so polite and full-of energy. She would always engage in conversations with her patients. Not that all the other nurses weren't lovely. She just stood out to me. I know it wasn't just me because so many people felt the same way; she was awarded the Daisy Award. The Daisy Award is when the hospital recognizes a nurse for all the work they have done. Anybody can nominate a nurse by adding their name to the Daisy Award nomination box.

I grew a special bond with Shelly during my second Zoladex shot. After I explained to her how terrible my first one was, she made sure that wasn't the case with her. She assured me that she would take her time and do her best to have a better outcome than the last nurse. After she used the Lidocaine, she offered me some ice. I held that on there while we waited the 15 mins. When she returned and tested the site, I didn't feel a thing, just a small amount of pressure. I thought to myself she has the magic touch. Ever since then she has been my favorite.

Now, I tell all the other nurses Shelly's remedy. Sometimes I'll even use my topical Lidocaine to numb it beforehand and that cuts down the time I have to let the injection of Lidocaine come to its full capability.

SUFFERING AND MANAGING SYMPTOMS

Some of the symptoms of chemotherapy can't be avoided; such as hair loss, loss of appetite, memory loss, aka chemo brain, altered taste buds, nail loss, dry skin, bruised skin, nausea, and pain caused by some of the symptoms. These are some of the symptoms I suffered. However, some symptoms can be avoided and or managed, such as mouth sores, which can cause an enormous amount of pain, and discourages one from eating. You can rinse with saline and salt a few times a day to prevent mouth sores. I rinsed in the beginning, but it got to be too much of a task, and I kept forgetting. So, eventually I stopped doing it all together. Luckily, I didn't suffer from mouth sores, but I did have a sore throat. The doctor prescribed a numbing magic mouthwash which is not available over the counter. The numbing is very temporary, and I mean 5 or 6 minutes.

Loss of appetite is manageable by ingesting, inhaling, or consuming cannabis. Some people say it even helps with nausea. However, it didn't give me any relief with that. On the other hand, it did help with my appetite when I smoked or ate an edible. Not too long after I would have the munchies. Even though the food still tasted nasty, I ate it. I wasn't aware of how happy I was eating until I couldn't enjoy it. Who would have known that taste buds were something to be grateful for?

As I mentioned before, eating something that you are not familiar with can partially help with your taste buds because there are no expectations. I spoke with Dr. Zimmerman about chemo brain/memory loss, and he suggested I start doing things that stimulated my brain, such as Sudoku and word puzzles. I would think "memory" would be an excellent game to play, as well. I don't believe there is anything that could help with nail loss. However, I did discover that press-on nails have come a long way. They are now available for your feet as well, and the adhesive is A1. For nausea, you could always ask the doctor for something else if what you have is not working. The most common drug is Zofran, and that didn't work for me. Ginger tea and candy also work for many people. I had a bit of relief with that remedy.

I later found that there were many side effects of Zoladex, including the many dark spots on my stomach after having to take the medicine from a needle the size of a screw. Some of the effects were the same as the chemo: vagina dryness, itching, discharge, an increase or decrease in sex drive, etc. I was concerned about the drought because I had never had that problem before having cancer, and I didn't want to experience it, mainly because I didn't like lubrication. I kept thinking that older adults used it. I never thought that it could be used to help people dealing with symptoms from medication. However, I never knew there could be symptoms that extreme.

Ask questions, get suggestions, and try new remedies.

I also suffered from "the phantom effect", which is a sensation in a limb or part of your body that has been amputated or the nerves are removed like in my case. When experienced, I feel something in my breast maybe, a tingle, an itch, or any type of sensation. When I spoke with my doctor, he said that it is typical and experienced more commonly than people would think. It would bother me when I had an itch but couldn't relieve it because I had no nerves there. It isn't painful or anything just a nuisance at times.

Some symptoms are never experienced. Some will come and go. But the most important thing I learned was to speak up. Ask questions, get suggestions, and try new remedies. What works for someone else may not work for you and vice versa. Also, keep a note pad to jot down symptoms, frequency, and severity. It is crucial to speak with your doctor about them. They may be able to prescribe something that can help you. In some cases, the symptoms you are suffering from can be a bad thing, so you always want to discuss things with your physician.

VICTORY!

I had concluded all my other treatments. Finally, it was my final day for treatment. My friends and family came along with me to my last treatment. Most of them waited patiently in the waiting room. The ones that came into the infusion room would have seen that I had a sign that said: "This is my last day of chemo."

After I was done, which was only 30 minutes, I went into the visiting room, where everyone was waiting for me. All the nurses that weren't busy at the time came out to watch me ring the bell. I was happy that all of them were there. But I waited for Shelly to wrap up with her patient, so she could witness me ringing the bell. She walked with me to the bell and said, "side to side, ok." I was so excited; I still tried to pull it, and there was nothing.

Moments later, I burst into tears. I couldn't believe it!

When I realized that I was doing it wrong, I switched my motion, and the sound of the bell rang. I heard the roars of cheers from everyone spectating in the visiting room. Moments later, I burst into tears. I couldn't believe it! That was the second time I cried tears of joy throughout this entire ordeal. I hugged my mom, dad, and my brother. Next, I hugged everyone that was there for me and even some people waiting to have their treatment. Then, I ran over to my lover and jumped in their arms. It seemed to be the warmest hug of them all.

I decided to have my port removed the same day. I didn't feel the need to have to come back another day for something I could do that day. Afterward, I wanted to do something small to celebrate completing all my treatments. Although I had

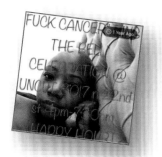

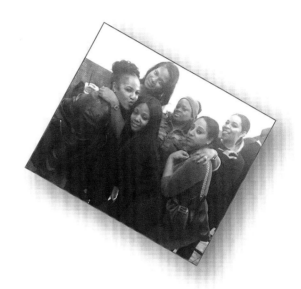

to take Tamoxifen once a day for the next ten years and continue to receive my Zoladex shot, I was cancer-free. It was time to get back to what I was doing before getting sick. But, before that, I wanted to have some legit fun; before I jumped into trying to be a responsible adult.

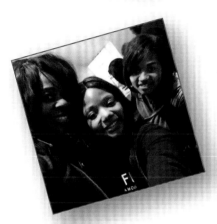

I chose a happy hour at one of the newest and probably the most beautiful hood bar in the city. My friends and family came to celebrate with me. But, as I said, it was something small during the week. So, I was happy with whoever could make it there to celebrate.

DATING

-N-

THINGS

Aye had been there through all my ups and downs. I shared things with her that I hadn't shared with anyone else. I could be myself with her. She made sure I was comfortable in my own skin. I didn't have to wear my unit, and she still would look at me like I was the baddest woman in the world. She never looked at me differently, her love was unconditional, pure, and never superficial. She knew how tired I was and how this had taken a toll on me.

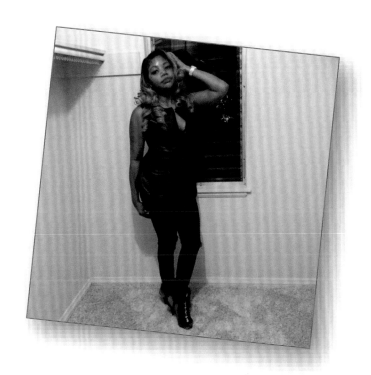

I met her towards the start of my aggressive treatments. I already knew of her, but "I met her, met her", if that makes any sense. I pulled her brother aside at a cookout and placed my bid. He passed it. Soon after, I knew it was successful because she was in my DM a.k.a direct message on Instagram. It was on. We went back and forth in the DM for a few days. To my surprise, her brother passed the bid but not the number. So, I slid her the number again. We were moving fast, from the DM to texting. It was looking good. After a few days of texting, we arranged to meet up.

Aye was tall and slim thick. Her skin was clear. Her nails were clean and neatly manicured, as well as her eyebrows. She wore two perfect braids to the back (I loved her hair like that). Her ears were pierced with two small diamond earrings. It was an immediate attraction during our date. It was more than physical, though; she had good conversation and good things going on in her life. Her heart was warm. It made me smile at some of the things she was doing for her community and people in need. We played table games while having ice cream. The vibes were lit. We shared many similar interests. However, Aye was very much a homebody, and I was the complete opposite.

Afterwards, we went our separate ways. We continued our communication via text. After realizing that neither of us had anything better to do, we hooked right back up. It had to be within the same hour that we left each other. We went to The Rec, and Aye taught me some stuff about basketball while we were shooting around. Then, we played Uno and sat outside until the wee hours of the morning, talking about any and everything. Before we parted ways, I asked what her relationship status was. Her response was, "I'm have a situation." Which was cool because I had someone I was talking to at the time as well. We were on the phone with each other before we pulled off.

"Ghost" was my babe. We weren't together, but that was my boo. However, our relationship was shifting a bit before I met Aye.

It was about a month later, and we were inseparable. Day in, until day out. Aye being a homebody made our bond ten times better. We were able to enjoy the things many people would call corny and boring. Her occupation allowed her to be absent during the summer and I was still recovering from surgery and off from work too. So, our days were consumed with each other. I completely forgot about the situation she mentioned previously. I think she almost did also. I was hardly spending any time with Ghost. No one else mattered when we were together.

We were crazy in love and completely obsessed with each other. She didn't give me any reason to be worried about anyone else. So, I didn't worry. I was safe, and my heart was being caressed with the softest touch. It had been so long since I felt this way.

Some days she would go get her hair braided or a few things out of the house, where she was living with her "situation". Still, I wasn't worried. Most of the time, she came right back outside afterward, and we would get back together. Even if we were doing things with our friends, we would bring the other right along. We were a unit.

Over time, I noticed things slowly beginning to change with her behavior. First, she would miss calls or wouldn't respond to texts for extended periods of time more than usual. Still, I wasn't alarmed. Soon after, she started going in her house for something and never coming back out. That's when I started to get on edge. But it didn't happen too often, so I still tried to remain calm. Her phone would ring more, and when she didn't answer the same name and number would continue to call over and over. I would see it on her phone if she left it near me or on the screen in the car if we were going somewhere. But, if she had her cellphone it hardly ever rang, or at least I didn't see it. When it did ring, I never asked any questions because I knew who was calling. After a while, I started to question her moves.

Here I was becoming jealous because she was still in love with the other woman.

I can recall one day it rang so much, and I told her to go ahead and answer. I understood her trying to be respectful and I felt like she wanted to answer. When the phone rang again, she pulled over and picked up her phone and excused herself. She was on the phone for so long I told her to take me back to my car. I had had enough at that point. So much for trying to be reasonable! Even though I loved her, she wasn't my girlfriend. I had to be mindful of that. However, things wouldn't have gone that way if it were me trying to answer my phone for someone else. But that's another story I want to save for another day.

I took some time to reflect on how our relationship was and where it was going. I thought about how Aye's phone had not been ringing. What was changing in their relationship to make her start calling the way she was? The dynamics of their relationship was changing; I felt it. Aye had to be feeding her something because she was on ice. Now, she was calling 100 mph. Something was going on, and I'm sure she knew it too.

Finally, after too long, I learned the truth. The "situation" Aye mentioned the first night was in fact a long-term, live-in family relationship of about five years. I know things end, so I wasn't worried about her "old fling" initially. Considering that she spent most nights out, I knew there had to be more than a little bit of trouble at home. Maybe at this point, I was naïve. I honestly thought that she would eventually break things off with her "old thing". I tried to convince myself that the other woman was trying to get back with Aye, and she wasn't interested. That had to be why she was calling. Weeks and months went by, and it never happened.

I had never been a jealous woman. Quite frankly, in this situation, she never gave me a reason to be. Here I was becoming jealous because she was still in love with the other woman. I couldn't believe it! I thought by now she would have been over her and she wasn't.

At one point, the phone would ring, and Aye wouldn't care to even look at it. Now, she was excusing herself to answer the phone (I had welcomed this into our relationship by allowing it the first time). She also pushed it so far to answer a few times while I was right there. I can recall lying in the bed and looking at this bi*** tell this woman she missed her. I couldn't believe she had the freaking nerve to say that in front of me. I was jealous. I can't lie. I didn't want her to miss her. Why would she miss her? I had no one to blame but myself. I had allowed it once and opened the door to this bs. It was too late. Meanwhile, I was developing a relationship with Aye's mother, who gave me the nickname, "Lil Tink Tink". We shared similar interests like cooking. She even shared her delicious crab recipe with me as we prepared it together in her kitchen.

On top of everything I had going on, I was now knowingly and willing, allowing myself to be the other woman for the first time in my life. My confidence and self-esteem were lower than usual because of everything I was going through. That was the excuse as to why I was accepting things I would have never allowed had I been in the right frame of mind.

I remember calling my dad to vent. I felt bad for continuing to deal with someone else's woman and possibly the reason for someone else's pain. He said it's natural to put your happiness before someone else's. However, I still didn't feel any better. I was sad, and I usually would keep things like this from my mom, but I confessed. I told her that I was the other woman. I'm sure she liked to think I was slow at this point. She said, "I didn't raise you that way. You have never been around anything of this nature because I would never want you to think that it's ok. It's not. And I don't ever want you to allow yourself to be one of someone's any options besides the only option." She was right. Either way, I couldn't leave her alone. Honestly, I didn't want to. I mean, I wanted to. But I didn't.

I still wanted to be with her every day. Not to mention, the sex that we were having was terrific. I can't lie because this is a transparent book. I still hope she isn't doing anyone how she was doing me….. AIN'T NO LOL BIHH!!

I remember the first time we had sex. It was so romantic. We were in a room full of rose petals and lit candles listening to Rihanna's Anti album. That was our favorite album. Ok. Ok. Ok. I was using my imagination. I got carried away. We were really in her car and coming from hanging out. I was grooving. So, I had the heart to do what I wanted to do that night (Mom, if you're reading this, skip a few paragraphs). I think she had to get out and get in the back seat. However, I just hopped in the back. If I don't remember anything else, I will FOREVER remember the sound of her belt unbuckling. It was terrifying. Anyway, I did what I saw them do on tv, I guess. It wasn't as bad as I anticipated. It was just very different from what would happen with a man though.

I was easily sexually satisfied with her. It had become so hard for me to climax because of the complications going on with my body. So much so, that after a while, I was able to stop faking my climaxes. Aye managed to learn my body as complicated as it was.

> I wanted to stay with her every night I could. Especially now because I was sharing her with someone else.

While dating Aye, I discovered a new symptom I was suffering from. Now that I was a lesbian, and I wasn't being penetrated. However, I had plenty of foreplay that would eventually cause me to bleed. But I didn't think much of it because I was going through so much. Anyway, when I did try to have sexual intercourse with Aye, I felt like I was losing my virginity. BABY!!!! THAT PAIN WAS SOMETHING ELSE!!!!!. Nonetheless, after trying to be penetrated more than once and having the same excruciating pain, we decided that we could maintain a healthy sexual relationship without it.

We were spending so many nights up all night sitting in the car. On the nights we couldn't stay at her mom's. I got tired of it. I wanted to stay with her every night I could. Especially now because I was sharing her with someone else. I needed all the time that was due to me. It was time for me to tell my mother about my sexual preference. She had no idea because I had been hiding dealing with women since before I even met Aye. I had no interest in men. My mom still had hopes that my ex and I would get back together. When I told her I was the other woman, I conveniently left out the part that I was also dating a woman.

I remember thinking, "Hopefully, my mom would be supportive, and I could have Aye over." I needed to face my mother with my truths.

ONLY CLOTHES BELONG IN THE CLOSET

We were in Atlantic City for her birthday. It was just my mother, my brother, and me. For some reason, there were a lot of LGBT people there. What a coincidence? She kept saying, "They all freaks, look at all these freaks, I ain't with the freaky-deeky stuff." I was screaming inside, knowing what I had to share with her. I felt like she was beating around the bush. She knew about me and was waiting for me to just come out with it.

I wasn't about to say anything yet. I wasn't strong enough. I needed some spinach. Where was Popeye when you needed him? The heart I had was now gone. I felt like a turtle; I just wanted to crawl back in my shell and tuck my head in tight. We enjoyed the rest of our time there, and I didn't speak a word of it. The next day we were in the house talking about how much fun we had the day before. Then, she started talking about how so many "freaks" were in Atlantic City.

I said, "Mom, I gotta tell you something."
Mom: "What? You a freak, like those people from yesterday?"
She began to laugh, but I remained quiet.
Me: "Yeah, mom."
Mom: "You're joking, right?"
Me: "No, mom, I'm a lesbian."
Mom: "Well, don't tell the people on my side of the family."

Then, she started talking about how so many "freaks" were in Atlantic City.

She chuckled again, but I think there was some authenticity behind that narrative. She seemed to be in denial. Next thing, she started talking about what she read in *Chicken Noodle Soup for Breast Cancer*. It mentioned how some women start affairs with women because they feel more confident and comfortable, and sometimes just perplexed during the life-altering ordeal. She also said that over time, the women went back to their original dating inclination. I never voiced to my mother that I had been dating women before being diagnosed. I just figured I would leave that part out. I wasn't volunteering too much info. Because I wanted to be honest, and I was staying with her, I told her. Otherwise, she would have found out when I married the girl of my dreams.

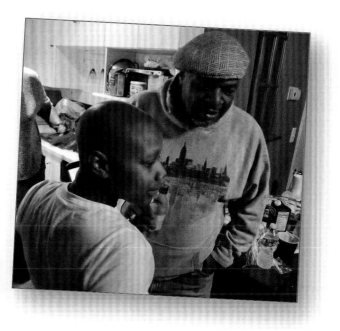

On the other hand, when I told my dad that I was a lesbian, he wasn't shocked, and I wasn't surprised. My dad and I have a cool relationship. I've been to plenty of strip clubs with him. I'm sure he knew what was up.

Getting back to the point, it was fun in the beginning with Aye, but then it began to cause me great heartache when Aye started to play the role of girlfriend with both her girlfriend and I (I can say "girlfriend" now but before I wouldn't have dared). Things took a turn for the worst when Aye's girlfriend found out about me and where I lived. As a result, trying to conceal that we still were together became a task. I never thought life as a side piece could be so damn complicated. I loved her but I was over being Tomb Raider at this point.

I'm sure her girlfriend knew what we were doing. She may have been in love, but she couldn't have been as naïve as I was. Aye was having it her way. But sooner or later it would catch up with her.

I witnessed a peculiar side of her I hadn't seen before. I noticed her bad anger issues when she started accusing me of dealing with other people. When, in fact, I didn't want to deal with anyone else. On the nights she couldn't come back outside, I would be upset and sad. I would stay home alone and on other nights hang out with my friends.

Aye tried me when she thought there was a two-for-one discount on the arguments. She thought that because she argued before she came out, that I was going to give her a pass. Nah, Sis! I'm mad too. So, let's have it!! Aye broke down crying one day because she was so frustrated. I guess it was finally catching up with her. It gave me a bit of joy to see her cry. Especially since I was crying all the time at this point. She was growing tired of the arguing and back and forth. I could sense the aggravation getting more severe each time. Until one day, she snapped, and it went further than words.

We were together and leaving Grand Lux Café in Cherry Hill. The plan was to stop pass Dior's house on the way home. I was connecting my Bluetooth to my car; Ghost was on the screen as one of the registered devices. Aye asked if I had been with her lately, and I explained that I hadn't seen her. I just hadn't erased her phone as a connected device. She didn't believe me. She sat quiet in the car the entire ride home and because that happened, I knew we wouldn't be stopping at Dior's house.

We pulled up to her mom's house and she mushed me on the way out of the car. For those who don't know what a mush is, it's when you place your hand on someone's head and push them. She assumed I was lying. However, I wasn't. But once she believed something, there was no changing her mind. I was taken back by the mush initially. I was mad, so mad. I couldn't believe her. She was still standing outside of the vehicle, and I hit her ass back. Then, I remembered I had Timberlands on, so I started kicking her and swinging at her. I pulled off furious.

After that, I didn't talk to her for a few days. I was mad and I needed to get over it. "It wasn't that big of a deal," I eventually thought. However, anyone putting their hands on me was a big deal. When I did talk to her, I explained that she was acting that way because of her guilty conscience. She apologized and admitted to overreacting. She promised not to do it again. She pacified me for a little while, and then it was back to the regularly scheduled program.

DÉJÀ
VU

Not long after completing all my treatments, I was applying lotion after a shower when I came across a dime size lump under my arm. It was right where I had my incision initially to biopsy my lymph node. I called the nurse, and she took a message. I waited to receive a call back from the doctor. I wasn't manic about it just a bit concerned. However, I still thought it was important enough to be persistent with trying to get in contact with Dr. Zimmerman to check it out.

I called back complaining about this lump for about two or three weeks. I wasn't that worried because I figured, what are the chances? I had taken preventative measures, and again this wasn't even breast tissue. It was tissue from my stomach. When Dr. Zimmerman finally called me back, I was scheduled to see him.

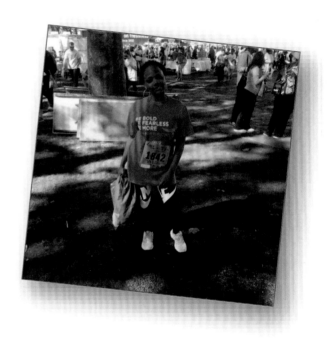

After doing a breast exam, he insisted I see my breast surgeon Dr. Li. When I talked to Dr. Li, I caught him up on what was going on, and I scheduled an appointment to see him. During my appointment, he did a breast exam. When he felt the lump, he applied pressure and asked me a few questions.

"Does it hurt?" he asked, "and how long has it been since you noticed it?" It wasn't painful and it had been a few weeks since I noticed it.

After everything was complete, he directed me not to worry. He said it was more than likely just fluid collecting from my surgery. I got a little nervous because I lied about how much fluid my drains were collecting because I wanted them out sooner than later. I messed up now, I thought.

He prescribed an ultrasound. When I got home, I went to sleep. My anxiety was getting the best of me and I needed to sleep it off. As anyone could imagine, I felt so uneasy. I heard my mom on the phone, "Yeah, they said it's just fluid." I still wasn't convinced.

✗

Waiting for results is never an easy thing to do, especially since I had cancerous cells the first time.

✗

The day of my ultrasound was just like the 30 I had prior. However, the techs didn't give me any "possible" or "maybes" this time. They just told me I would hear from the doctor when the results came in, which would be in the next few days. Waiting for results is never an easy thing to do, especially since I had cancerous cells the first time. So, I tried to keep myself busy doing my favorite hobbies. I also tried to believe there was no way that I could have cancer again. But one can never be too sure.

I was at work a few days later when I finally received the call from Dr. Li. He told me he had some concerns about what he thought was fluid, and he wanted me to have further testing. Then, he insisted that I have a biopsy done as soon as possible.

I was scheduled for a biopsy again! The biopsy was just like any of the other ones I had already had. However, I grew more anxious and curious as to what it could be causing this lump.

Waiting for the results was the most challenging because Dr. Li was growing concerned and I too, was becoming even more interested. Everyone was telling me to have faith. I was sick just thinking about having to go through it all over again.

I was at work when I finally received a call back from Dr. Li with the results…

The story isn't over. Stay tuned for Book Two, ***The Cancer Slayer, The Rematch.***

EPILOGUE

Whenever I feel like I am at my lowest, or not taking advantage of my life, or maybe even being ungrateful for still being here, things happen. Again, not that I am the most spiritual person, but in some cases, I feel like things happen to give me a reminder or a sign rather than a coincidence. I know this is cliché, but I'll say it anyway, **"everything happens for a reason".** People come into your life for a reason. This is a way to look at things more positively. Here are some of the people that came into my life and helped me out along the way:

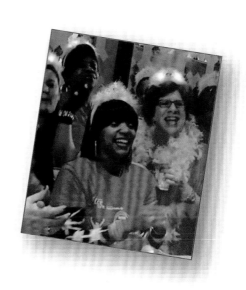

Sophia Grace

I remember speaking with Lynn in the group chat, and she told us that Sophia wasn't feeling well. Everyone checked on Sophia and her family daily to make sure they were okay. However, after a few days, she hadn't improved. So, Lynn took her to the hospital. Soon after, we found out she had Leukemia. We were all devastated. It's always sad to find out that someone has cancer. It hits a lot harder when it is a child, though.

Sophia was a beautiful five-year-old. She had long, pretty hair that came all the way down to her back. Every time I would come to see her mom, she would be upset because she felt like I was her company. Probably because we were the same size. She was so full of energy at that age.

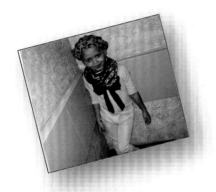

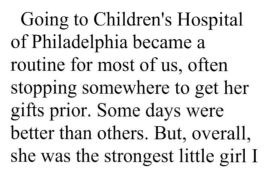

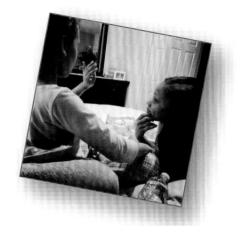

Going to Children's Hospital of Philadelphia became a routine for most of us, often stopping somewhere to get her gifts prior. Some days were better than others. But, overall, she was the strongest little girl I knew. When her hair began to fall out, she was upset. But she didn't let it get the best of her. She embraced her new look just as a princess should. I saw her push through. The best part of such a bad time for her was, every day, she looked forward to what we were bringing her. Every day was Christmas.

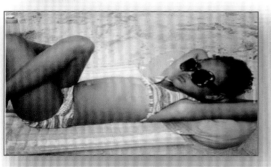

It brought many of us joy to see her happy. She suffered from all the common symptoms, but she fought like a champ. She even wanted to go to school. Little did I know this experience was preparing me for later. Sophia is now 12 years old and has been cancer free for 7 years!

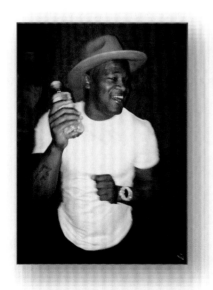

Jamal

Around the time I was diagnosed, a friend of mine, Jamal announced that he had brain cancer. I was traumatized. I couldn't believe that someone that I knew would be going through this with me. Jamal wasn't speaking of or posting much about his condition on social media. Mal and I communicated back and forth from time to time via direct message on Instagram. When I did talk to him, he would always tell me how well he was doing with everything. I remember mentioning to him that he didn't post enough, and I wanted him to do more interacting. I told him how much it helped me. I thought that it might help him to talk about it.

He assured me that he was just fine watching my posts. He said, "Nah, Dom you post for all of us," referring to the cancer warriors who didn't share their story.

Time went on, and Jamal or what most of us called him, Mal, posted a few times. From what I understood, Mal spent a lot of time in the hospital. His cancer was considered very severe. I would ask him if he was ok and if he needed anything, and he would always

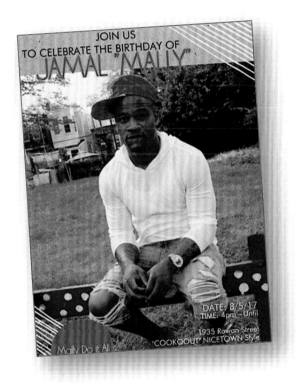

decline. I made sure he always confirmed that he was doing fine, and his health was improving or steady. I was happy to hear that a fellow warrior was beating the odds. I can't explain it anymore besides saying it's motivating as crap!

Months passed, and our regular talks had turned into maybe once a month if that. Then, I received a call from Liah. She told me that Jamal wasn't doing good. I immediately went to see him. I needed to lay my eyes on him. I couldn't believe that he wasn't doing well. All this time, he was doing ok, or so he said.

When I arrived, he looked like himself. He had some swelling in his head due to the tumor. However, he still was able to talk and comprehend. I asked him, "Mal, why didn't you tell me that your health was declining?" He replied, "Dom, my health never was improving. I would apologize but, I would be lying. The truth is, I didn't want to discourage you during your battle."

I was speechless. What Jamal had done was such a selfless act. I couldn't even be upset with him. As I admired such a strong man, trying to fight back my tears, I was interrupted by a tech who was taking him away for some scans. He told me he didn't need anything before he left the room. I promised to return to see him in two days. I couldn't come back the next day because I had my appointments and I had to work the following day.

Two days later, I was on my way to the hospital. I needed his last name again, so I called Liah and asked her for the room number. That's when she told me he had passed not too long before then. I couldn't believe that I never even made it back to see him. I can't express how discouraging it is to watch people pass away one by one from cancer while you're fighting cancer.

It made me question what I was doing all of it for anyway? What if I fight all this time, and I still die?

At Jamal's Jenazah, it is customary to not cry loudly or sob near the body. In his Muslim community, Jamal would be punished for it in the afterlife. That only made things worse for those of us who were there to pay our respects and were not followers of Islam. As I watched the men shovel the dirt over his body, my mind drifted off to my funeral. How things would go and how sad people would be. I figured I would be better off getting cremated.

Debbie Dawson

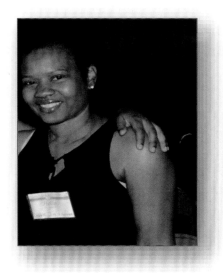

Nor introduced me to Ms. Debbie. She was a friend of his, and she had just been diagnosed with breast cancer for the third time. She was also related to Penelope. When we decided to link up, I took her to one of my favorite restaurants here in the city, Sampan. We talked and shared so many similar interests. Then we discussed and compared our diagnosis and treatment plans.

Ms. Debbie couldn't work during her treatments. Unlike me, she was in great pain while fighting. Since Ms. Debbie was tired of being treated at the hospitals and it not being successful, she decided to try to treat it holistically. She was using black salve as an alternative treatment for cancer. Black salve is an herbal cure for cancer. It's placed on the skin and is supposed to force the impurities to come through the skin. I learned that it is illegal to sell as an alternative treatment for cancer almost all over the world. Along with the black salve, she was having oxygen and vitamin C treatments.

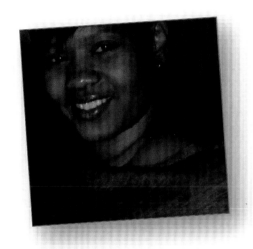

The vitamin C treatments were every other day and $120 per injection. The oxygen treatments were once a week and $400 per session. Although these procedures were pricey, they were not being given by doctors or nurses who were state bound certified. She told me that her daughter had been doing some research on holistic therapies. She believed that treating it this way was the best option for her, especially since she had not been successful fighting the disease traditionally.

Considering how pricey this treatment was, I assumed she was getting assistance from her insurance company. However, she informed me that she had to pay for these treatments out of pocket. I couldn't believe what I was hearing. After doing the math, it was roughly over $3000 a month. We finished up our date, hugged, and promised to keep in touch.

When I talked to her again, we reflected on our initial conversation and how she was handling the pain. I recalled while we were together that she had a pillow under her arm. However, I figured it had to do with her diagnosis and didn't ask any questions. I was now learning that she used the pillow to avoid putting pressure on the tumor that was under her arm. She asked me if I had a weak stomach, I told her at times. She followed with a picture of how her tumor looked from applying the black salve. It appeared to be terribly painful. The skin that once covered the tumor was almost completely gone and exposed her flesh. It was probably the

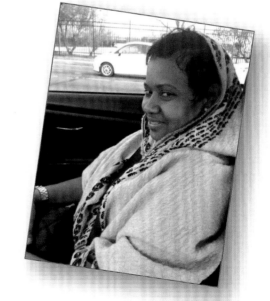

size of a baby's head. I shared with her how strong I thought she was. She was going through so much and still trying to remain positive.

Overtime we kept in touch and would text and call to check on each other. I would always suggest that she at least go to see a doctor to see what stage her cancer had progressed to. That went on for months. Until she finally went. They told her she was now staged 4.

By that time, she had given up using the alternative treatments and decided she would try chemotherapy again. Not long after she started her treatments, she stated that she was tired, and she wasn't going to fight it anymore. I told her I would support any of her choices. I also told her that if anyone questioned her decisions, she should waste no time trying to explain anything to them.

Our calls grew further apart. About two months went by, and I hadn't heard from Ms. Debbie. I texted her and told her I was checking on her. A few days went by after that, and I still hadn't heard from her. So, I called her and her phone was disconnected. I spoke with Nor and told him I was having trouble reaching her. I asked him to see if he could try to get in touch with her for me. His attempts were unsuccessful, as well.

Next, I reached out to P. Ms. Debbie was like an aunt to her. She hadn't heard from her either and would ask around to have her call me.

When P did get back to me, it was news I wasn't prepared to receive. Ms. Debbie had succumbed to the disease. She didn't have any further information regarding the funeral or anything at that time. I couldn't believe she had passed. I didn't even know her health had become terminal.

I was saddened by the news I had received. I was more upset because I knew she had stage four cancer, but I thought she would survive much longer. I was looking forward to having another date with her. Her health had been declining over time. Unfortunately, another cancer warrior had passed, and again I wasn't even able to say goodbye.

Melvin & Pam

After my cousin Melvin's death, I learned that he had stomach cancer but died of other complications. It was an eye-opener, but at his burial, I saw someone's headstone right above his site. It had the breast cancer ribbons on it, so of course, it caught my eye. While reading, the headstone said she fought a good fight. Then, I saw the date, March 2018. I read the name Pamela, and my knees got weak.

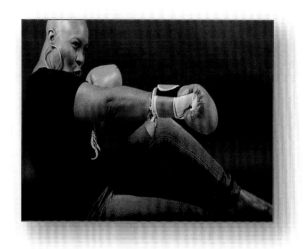

Pam was a woman I met on social media. She wrote to me often. She was like my Instagram, mom. Although I never met her, we developed a relationship. She would contact me and check on me periodically, and I would do the same. I was having a rough time with my emotions and deactivated my page for a while. A few weeks later, when I logged back in, I learned of Ms. Pam's passing. Again, my heart filled with uncertainty. I didn't know what my fate would be.

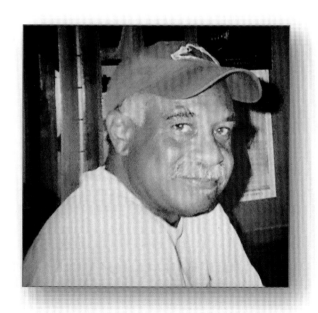

What are the chances that I would be standing in front of Ms. Pam's gravesite? I had never been in a cemetery and stumbled upon someone's headstone I knew. NEVER! It was a heartbreaking moment. I felt like I had just got the news all over again and I was instantly overwhelmed with emotions and had to excuse myself from the remainder of the service. I was on an emotional rollercoaster, but most of all, grateful to be alive and to have things to look forward to. At that moment, I knew there were more changes I needed to make in my life to get back to my happy place.

MEMORIES

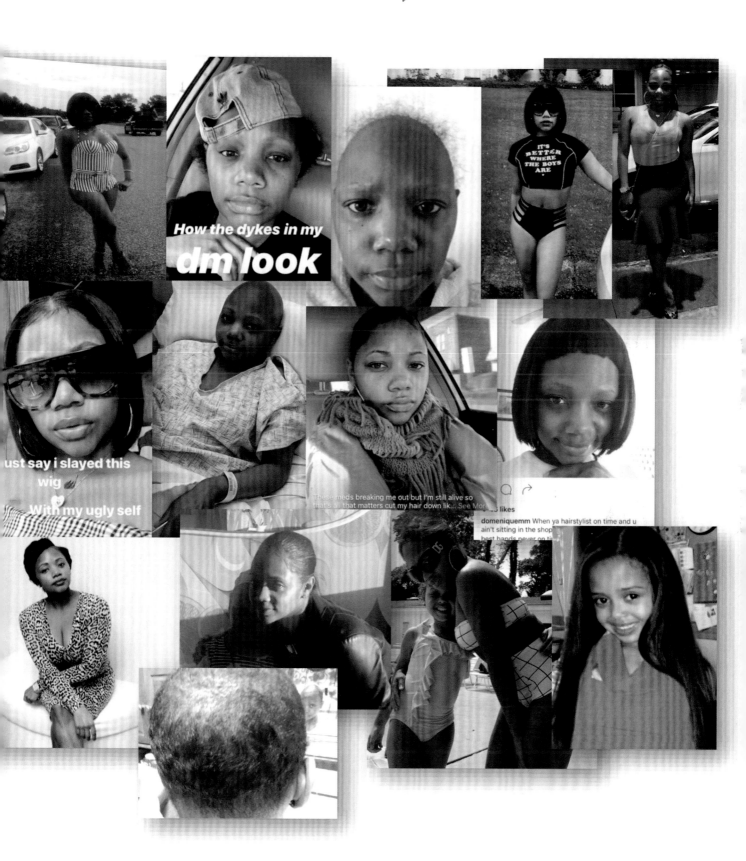

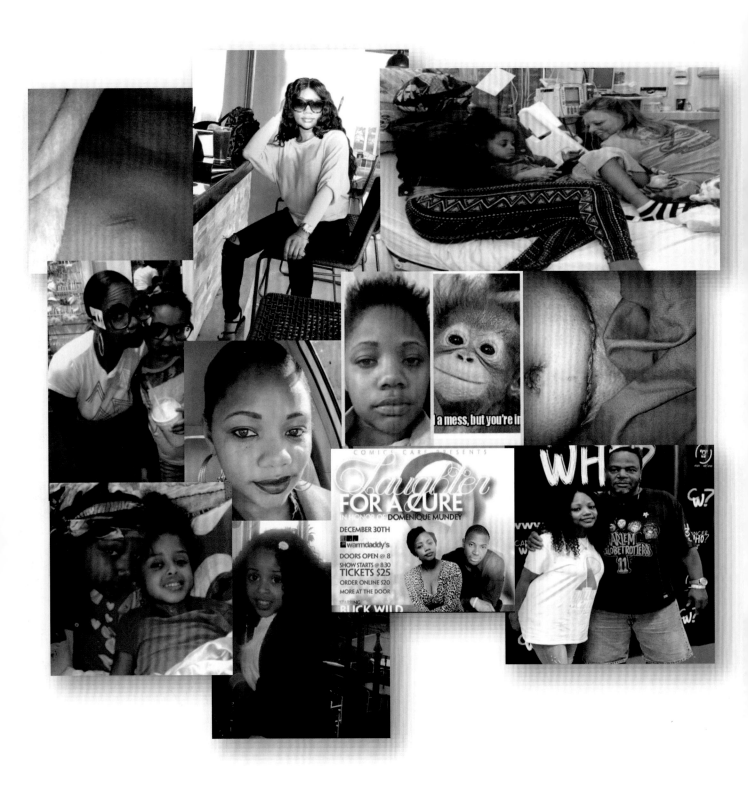

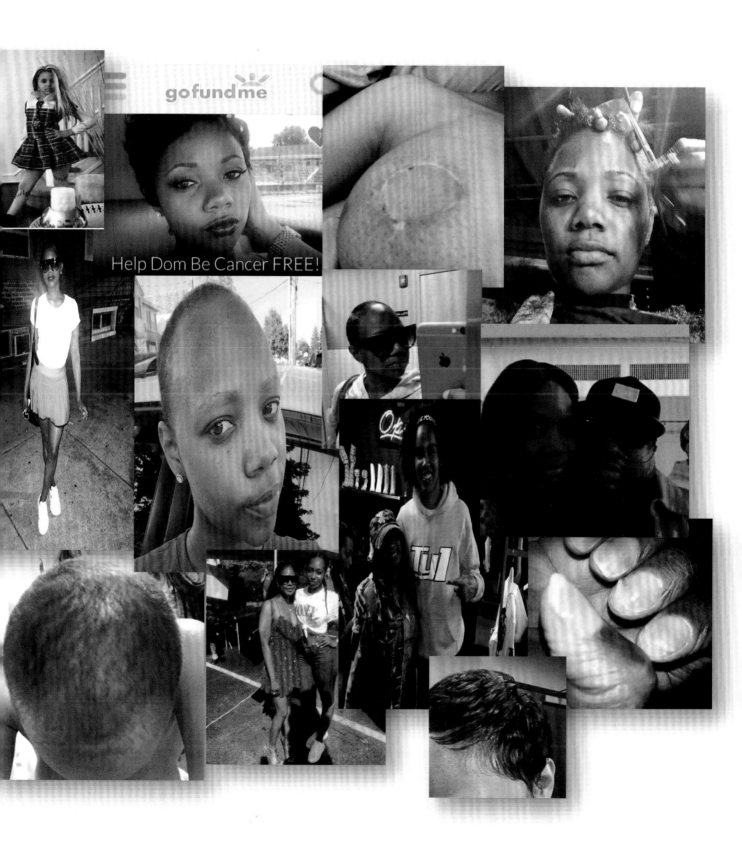

In Loving Memory of

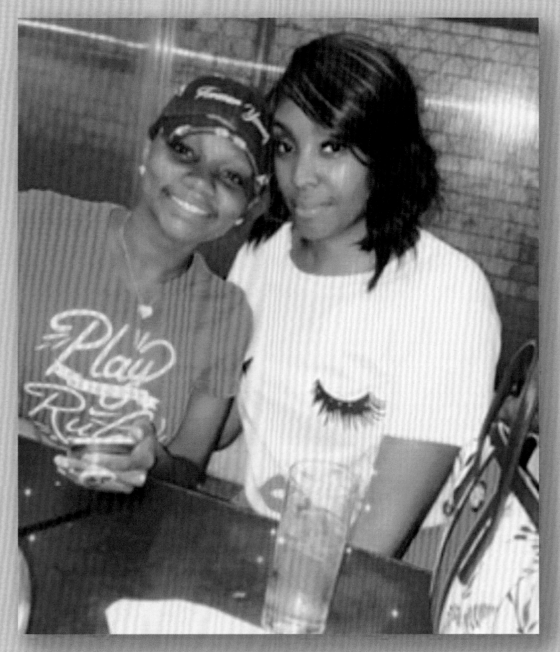

Jasmine Witherspoon

In Loving Memory of

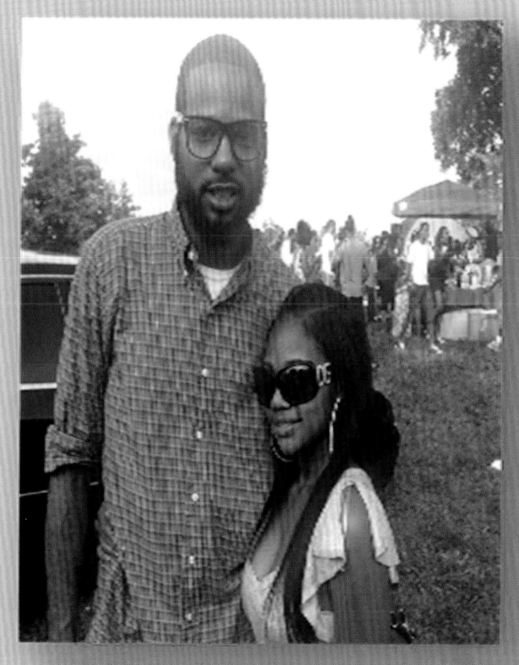

Thomas English Jr,